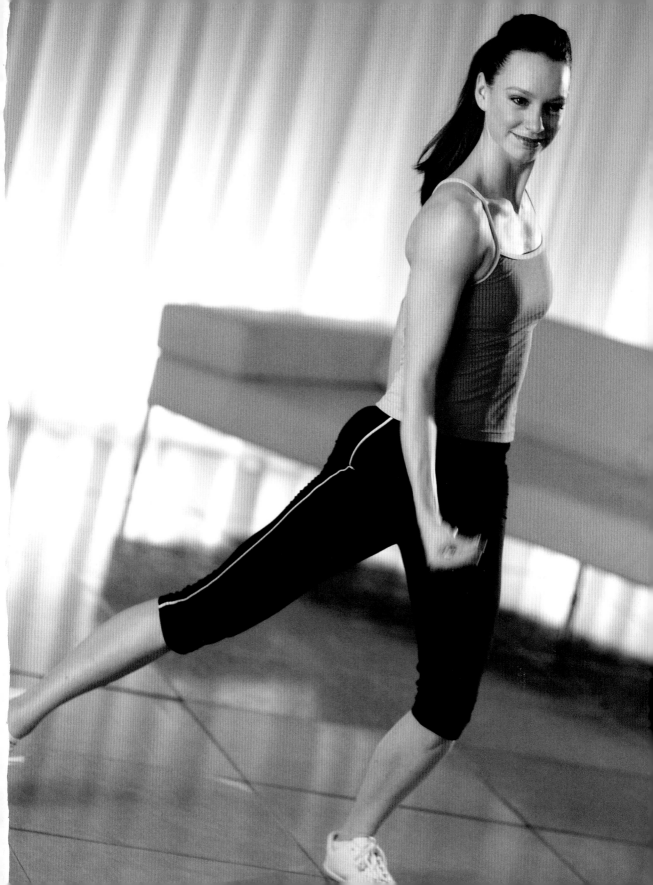

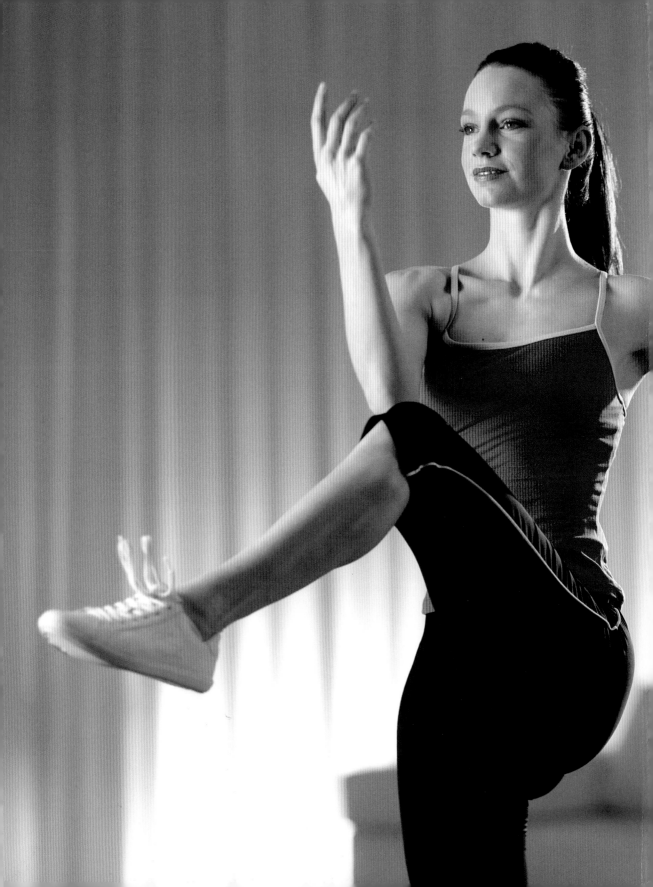

>> **15** minute

dance

workout

Caron Bosler

London, New York, Melbourne, Munich, and Delhi

Project Editor Hilary Mandleberg
Project Art Editor Anne Fisher
Project Assistant Andrew Roff
Senior Editor Jennifer Latham
US Editor Christy Lusiak
Senior Art Editor Susan Downing
Managing Editor Dawn Henderson
Managing Art Editor Christine Keilty
Art Director Peter Luff
Publishing Director Mary-Clare Jerram
Stills Photography Ruth Jenkinson
DTP Designer Sonia Charbonnier
Production Controller Alice Holloway
Production Editor Luca Frassinetti

DVD produced for Dorling Kindersley by
Chrome Productions www.chromeproductions.com
Director Gez Medinger
Producer Hannah Chandler
DOP Benedict Spence
Camera Benedict Spence, Joe McNally
Production Assistant Irene Maffei
Grip Terry Williams
Gaffer Jonathan Spencer
Music Chad Hobson / Scott Shields / Felix Erskine
Hair and Makeup Victoria Barnes
Voiceover Caron Bosler
Voiceover Recording Ben Jones

First American Edition, 2009

Published in the United States by
DK Publishing
375 Hudson Street
New York, New York 10014

09 10 11   10 9 8 7 6 5 4 3 2 1

AD408—January 09

Published in Great Britain by Dorling Kindersley Limited.
A catalog record for this book is available from the Library
of Congress.

ISBN 978-0-7566-4202-0

DK books are available at special
discounts when purchased in bulk
for sales promotions, premiums,
fund-raising, or educational use.
For details, contact: DK Publishing
Special Markets, 375 Hudson Street,
New York, New York 10014 or
SpecialSales@dk.com.

Health warning
All participants in fitness activities must assume the
responsibility for their own actions and safety. If you have
any health problems or medical conditions, consult with
your doctor before undertaking any of the activities set
out in this book. The information contained in this book
cannot replace sound judgment and good decision
making which can help reduce the risk of injury.

Printed and bound in China by Sheck Wah Tong
Printing Press Ltd.

Discover more at
www.dk.com

contents

>> **author** foreword

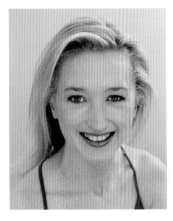

Like most girls in Texas, I started dance class at the age of 12, to appease a nagging mother who was secretly praying that I would learn to walk straight with a little more grace than a bulldozer. To her surprise, I loved it. The annual dance recital is the highlight of most dance schools, and before I left for North Carolina School of the Arts at 15 years old to study dance, I went out with a bang. On stage, first piece, collision with a sound box, head injury, eight stitches. The ambulance crew came down the center aisle...

While learning to avoid sound boxes in high school, I started working in gyms to help support myself while dancing. After that, I never stopped studying. I continued my journey northward and studied dance in college at The State University of New York at Purchase. In 1992, I was a freshman, and traded free certification in the Pilates Method for free labor. A year and a half later, I knew I'd hit it big time when I was teaching Pilates for $12 an hour. What I didn't know, and am happy to say, was that my college job would become my life. Teaching health and fitness proved to be a wonderful way to support myself while on scholarship with The Merce Cunningham Dance Company in New York and throughout my Masters in Dance at The Laban Centre, London.

Now I have moved to London, and although I quit dancing professionally at 28 years old, dance is still at the heart of everything I teach and do. The principles I learned when studying dance—posture, length, elongation, moving from your core, poise, grace, fluidity, and style—have transcended the classroom and become part of my everyday life. They can be part of yours, too.

I incorporate all those principles in the private fitness lessons I have given over the last 10 years. This time has been a truly unique and wonderful experience. The benefit of teaching people in their own homes is that you can really get to know them and get to the root of what will motivate them. Part of that motivation lies in ensuring that they are having fun during the lesson. If the client is not enjoying exercising, he or she won't do it again.

The downside to private training is that you are limited by the hours in a day and the number of people you can meet in that time. Working on this project is my way of trying to spread some of the fun—and my passion for dance—just a little bit further. The most important thing I would like anyone to get out of these workouts is the sheer joy of dancing. Sweating, having a fit body, plenty of stamina, and flexibility come in just a touch below...

The best way to enjoy these dance workouts is to allow yourself the freedom to play. Doing this without self-judgment is all part of the joy of learning something new. So start by committing to make time for yourself to learn this new skill. You will feel more positive and uplifted, knowing you are doing something, every day, that benefits your heart, lungs, body, and mind. This is my hope—for anyone who wants to get and stay in shape.

>> **how to use** this book

Each of the four 15-minute dance programs in this book offers a complete, aerobically structured workout (see p14). Take time to study the exercises in detail and familiarize yourself with each step. Use the gatefold summary as a quick reminder.

Each of the dance programs can be done at a beginner, intermediate, or advanced pace. You do not have to do them in any particular order—just start with the one you like the look of best.

The accompanying DVD demonstrates all four programs. Before starting each dance, read through the workout in the book so that you are familiar with what lies ahead, and what aspects to focus on. For example, the ballet workout highlights soft, beautiful arms, while the salsa workout centers on the movement of the hips.

The DVD offers a mirror image for you to follow along with, just as you would mirror the teacher in a dance class. The voice-over helps to reinforce the DVD, by giving the name of each movement along with telling you which leg you should be using. As you watch the DVD, page references to the book flash up on the screen. Refer to these for more detailed instruction. The insets in the book will help remind you of the step you have recently done and to which you are about to add a variation. The annotations give you tips on proper positioning or what to watch out for in each movement.

Finally, throughout the book, one repetition, or rep, refers to repeating a move to both right and left.

The gatefolds
These show each dance workout from beginning to end. Once you've watched the DVD and examined each move, use the gatefolds as a quick reference. The more familiar you are with each workout, the better you will perform them.

Safety issues
Be sure to get clearance from your healthcare provider prior to beginning any exercise program. The advice and exercises here are not intended to be a substitute for individual medical help. Your medical specialist may recommend preparatory exercises especially tailored to your needs.

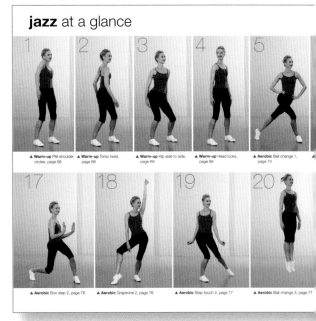

jazz at a glance

▲ **Warm-up** Plié shoulder circles, page 68 ▲ **Warm-up** Torso twist, page 68 ▲ **Warm-up** Hip side to side, page 69 ▲ **Warm-up** Head looks, page 69 ▲ **Aerobic** Ball change 1,
page 70

▲ **Aerobic** Box step 2, page 76 ▲ **Aerobic** Grapevine 2, page 76 ▲ **Aerobic** Step touch 2, page 77 ▲ **Aerobic** Ball change 3, page 77

The gatefold gives you a comprehensive demonstration of the entire workout—an easy reference to make your practice quick and simple.

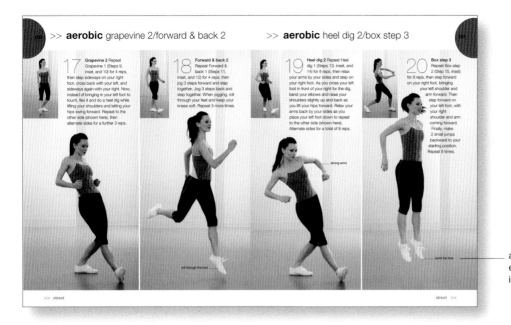

>> **aerobic** grapevine 2/forward & back 2   >> **aerobic** heel dig 2/box step 3

17 Grapevine 2 Repeat Grapevine 1 (Steps 9, inset, and 10) for 4 reps, then step sideways on your right foot, cross back with your left, and sideways again with your right. Now, instead of bringing in your left foot to touch, flex it and do a heel dig while lifting your shoulders and letting your hips swing forward. Repeat to the other side (shown here), then alternate sides for a further 3 reps.

18 Forward & back 2 Repeat Forward & back 1 (Steps 11, inset, and 12) for 4 reps, then jog 3 steps forward and step together. Jog 3 steps back and step together. When jogging, roll through your feet and keep your knees soft. Repeat 3 more times.

19 Heel dig 2 Repeat Heel dig 1 (Steps 13, inset, and 14) for 8 reps, then relax your arms by your sides and step on your right foot. As you cross your left foot in front of your right for the dig, bend your elbows and raise your shoulders slightly up and back as you lift your hips forward. Relax your arms back by your sides as you place your left foot down to repeat to the other side (shown here). Alternate sides for a total of 8 reps.

20 Box step 3 Repeat Box step 2 (Step 15, inset) for 8 reps, then step forward on your right foot, bringing your left shoulder and arm forward. Then step forward on your left foot, with your right shoulder and arm coming forward. Finally, make 2 small jumps backward to your starting position. Repeat 8 times.

strong arms

roll through the foot

point the toes

annotations provide extra cues, tips, and insights

>> street   street >>

Step-by-step pages The inset photograph at the upper left gives you the previous variation of the movement, unless stated otherwise. The large photograph shows you the next level of the movement.

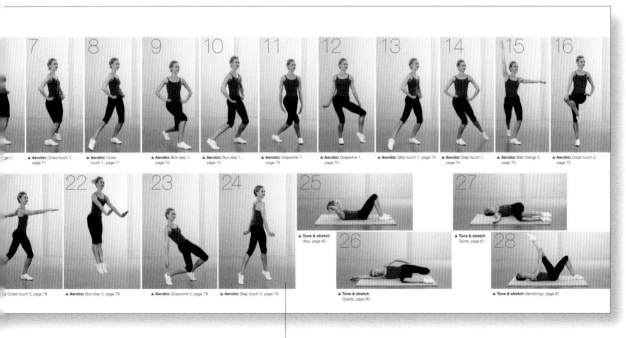

7   8   9   10   11   12   13   14   15   16

▲ Aerobic Cross touch 1, page 71   ▲ Aerobic Cross touch 1, page 71   ▲ Aerobic Box step 1, page 72   ▲ Aerobic Box step 1, page 72   ▲ Aerobic Grapevine 1, page 73   ▲ Aerobic Grapevine 1, page 73   ▲ Aerobic Step touch 1, page 74   ▲ Aerobic Step touch 1, page 74   ▲ Aerobic Ball change 2, page 75   ▲ Aerobic Cross touch 2, page 75

22   23   24   25   27

▲ Aerobic Cross touch 3, page 78   ▲ Aerobic Box step 3, page 78   ▲ Aerobic Grapevine 3, page 79   ▲ Aerobic Step touch 3, page 79

▲ Tone & stretch Abs, page 80   ▲ Tone & stretch Spine, page 81

26   28

▲ Tone & stretch Quads, page 80   ▲ Tone & stretch Hamstrings, page 81

the gatefold shows all the main steps of the sequence

>> **exercise** and posture

Exercise benefits your mind as well as your body. It makes you feel more energized and better prepared for whatever life throws at you. And, if you cultivate good postural habits, you will not only see the benefits in your everyday movements, but you'll start to look and feel better too.

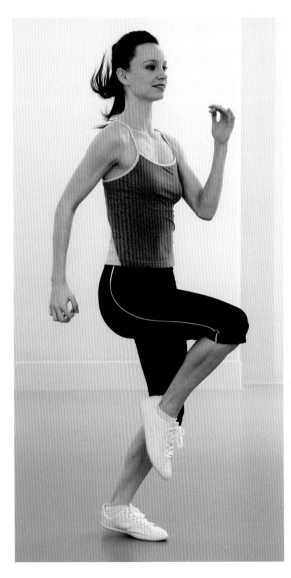

Aerobic, or cardiovascular, exercise simply means any form of exercise that keeps the heart rate high over a sustained period of time. Aerobic literally means "with oxygen." By increasing the heart rate and strengthening the heart (see p14) and lungs, the body is able to use oxygen more efficiently. The system known as "aerobic exercise" was first developed in 1968 by Dr. Kenneth H. Cooper in San Antonio, Texas. It originally consisted of exercises such as cycling, running, and swimming, but from those simple beginnings arose the aerobics exercise phenomenon we know today.

The "Talk Test"

Always work within safe limits when exercising. The simplest way of checking is to use the "Talk Test." Quite simply, if you can talk comfortably while you are exercising, your heart rate is functioning within a safe range. If you are feeling breathless or uncomfortable, you should stop.

Correct posture

Correct posture and alignment are important not only when exercising, but in your daily life as well. Walking, standing, carrying heavy objects, or holding briefcases all take their toll on the spine. With just a little effort, you can have perfect posture and a healthy spine throughout your life.

Continuous aerobic exercise enhances the production of serotonin, a neurotransmitter with effects on the brain that include mood elevation.

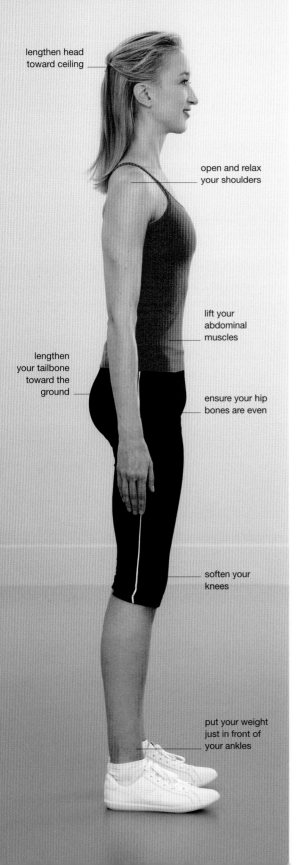

lengthen head
toward ceiling

open and relax
your shoulders

lift your
abdominal
muscles

lengthen
your tailbone
toward the
ground

ensure your hip
bones are even

soften your
knees

put your weight
just in front of
your ankles

Practice standing correctly every day, and you will see the benefits in no time. A good time to practice is in the morning while you are brushing your teeth in front of the mirror. Stand with your feet hip-width apart and parallel to each other. Make sure your weight is evenly distributed between your feet. Rock slightly forward and back on your toes and ankles. You want to settle your weight slightly in front of your ankles. Your knees should be soft and never locked. Your hip bones should be even—check that they are not tilted to one side or the other—and your tailbone should be lengthening toward the ground. Lift your abdominal muscles and lengthen your head up toward the ceiling. Think of your shoulders as open and relaxed. Envision a vertical line straight from the top of your ear and through the middle of your shoulder, hip, knee, and ankle.

Get used to this feeling, and, as you carry on with your everyday life, try to think about how you are standing from time to time. Keep that awareness when sitting, too, making sure that your head and abs are lifting, and that your shoulders are open.

Correct posture and alignment are essential in preventing lower-back pain. By pulling in the abdominal muscles, pressure is taken off the lower back.

>> **benefits** of aerobic exercise

- **Reduces** the risk of heart disease, diabetes, and other diseases
- **Helps** weight loss
- **Improves** metabolism
- **Strengthens** the heart
- **Lowers** the resting heart rate, which means your heart does not have to work as hard to pump blood around your body
- **Increases** the body's ability to use oxygen more efficiently and so burn fat faster
- **Decreases** stress levels

>> **dance** into fitness

When you practice dance, you will notice an improvement in poise, grace, alignment, and coordination, as well as a better understanding of rhythm, an improvement in your memory, increased self-esteem, and a greater appreciation of music. There are many other benefits, too.

In addition to giving you a great workout and improving your balance, dance will give you elongated, well-defined, well-toned muscles and a strong, sculpted body. It stretches and strengthens the muscles, but works the body very differently than lifting heavy weights in the gym, which builds bulk and shortens the muscles. Dance is also great for increasing the flexibility of the spine, hips, and other joints. And if that weren't enough, it also gives you the greater self-awareness you need to improve your posture and alignment.

Most postural problems occur through lack of awareness and laziness. By introducing dance into your life, you will become more aware of the

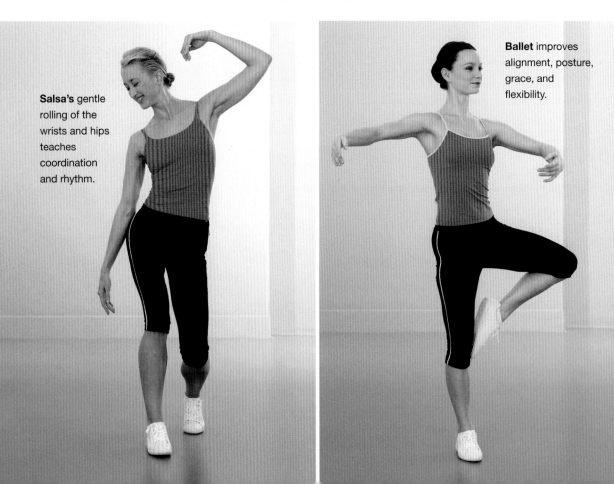

Salsa's gentle rolling of the wrists and hips teaches coordination and rhythm.

Ballet improves alignment, posture, grace, and flexibility.

position of your head, neck, and shoulders in relation to the rest of your body (see pp10–11), and that is the first step on the road to correction.

Dance as an aerobic activity

Unfortunately, because of the way a dance class is usually structured, dance is not usually considered to be an aerobic activity. Normally, a ballet teacher, for example, will stop the class each time he or she wants to show a sequence at the barre or when teaching floor work. True aerobic activity must be continuous, so this type of dance class will not offer you an aerobic workout.

My four workouts give you the best of both worlds: A combination of aerobics and dance. And, they can be enjoyed in optimal time—just 15 minutes! What is more, each one can be tailored to beginner, intermediate, or advanced levels. You don't have to do them in a specific order: Just start with your favorite dance style.

Why these dance styles?

In my choice of dance styles for this project, I have tried to reflect something of the vast range of popular dance genres. I have chosen from both mainstream popular dance culture and from dance as a classical art form. As you learn a few moves from classical ballet, I hope you will gain a greater understanding and appreciation of that style of dance. The tone and movements of the jazz workout are reminiscent of Bob Fosse and the Broadway musical. Salsa, with its gentle rolling of the hips, has a sultry Latin-American mood, while the street workout has an earthy, grounded feel. One dance genre might appeal to you more than another, but trying them all can be lots of fun.

The movements are really easy to pick up. Always learn the feet first, then add the arms, and, when you are feeling confident, add the shoulders and hips. Don't forget to have fun and to add your own personal style to the steps.

Jazz enhances coordination, balance, and muscle tone through powerful, sharp-angled movements.

Street improves rhythm and coordination and encourages diversity of movement.

>> **the structure** of a workout

Usually, when you go to an aerobics class, you will notice that the exercise you do has three distinct sections. First there is the warm-up, then the aerobic section, and finally, a toning and stretching section. These dance workouts are structured in exactly the same way.

The warm-up does exactly what you would imagine. It warms up the body and mobilizes the joints and muscles in preparation for the exercise that follows. If you walked into class without warming up and went straight into jumping, you could seriously injure yourself. By performing some light stretches as a warm-up, you open the joints, increase their range of motion, and are getting the body ready for more active movement.

The aerobic section

The aerobic section is the longest section of any aerobics class. It is designed to exercise your heart. The heart is a muscle and, just like other muscles, responds well to exercise. Your heart rate is the number of times your heart beats, or contracts, per minute. Doing aerobic exercise gently increases the number of beats per minute, raising the heart rate, and strengthening the heart. The aerobic curve is a term used to describe how, during aerobic exercise, your heart rate is gently increased, sustained, and then brought back down to your resting heart rate.

In this book and DVD, each dance workout consists of five basic movements (Level 1). You start by performing these, then they are developed aerobically in various ways, such as by the addition of an arm movement, or by a deeper bend of the knees, or by traveling the movement through space (Level 2). At the peak of the aerobic curve, jumping movements are usually involved (Level 3). If you find these uncomfortable, then perhaps you are not yet

Aerobic exercise such as jogging, skipping, and cycling strengthens and improves the efficiency of the heart and lungs.

ready for them. Don't worry, though, because you can still get a great workout simply by performing the movements without doing the jumps.

Finally, to bring the heart rate back to your resting heart rate, you reverse all the movements, first taking out all the jumps, then taking out the second developments. You finish as you started, by performing the five basic movements on their own.

Toning and stretching

After the aerobic portion of the workout, you will then lie down on a mat to do some toning and stretching. Toning strengthens individual muscles or groups of muscles without building bulk. Examples of some toning exercises are abdominal exercises or light push-ups. By doing a few abdominal exercises every day, you can increase the strength of these core muscles. The result will be strong abdominal muscles that help support the spine and ease lower-back pain.

While strengthening helps to tone the muscles, stretching keeps the muscles and joints supple. In these workouts, you may, for example, end up doing a hamstring stretch or a hip stretch.

The photographs below show an example of a simple toning exercise.

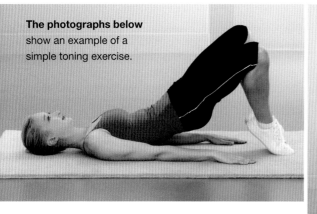

Step 1 Start with your knees bent, feet flat on the floor and together. Now roll your pelvis off the floor, one vertebra at a time, lifting your heels up and inhaling as you slowly open your knees.

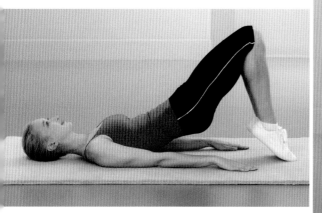

Step 2 As you exhale, squeeze your knees together. This exercise strengthens and tones the muscles of the hamstrings, inner thighs, and calves.

You can stretch specific muscles. The inset photograph shows stretching the front of the thigh by lengthening the muscles in the quadriceps. The main photograph shows how to stretch the calf muscle.

keep the shoulders open and relaxed

make sure the toes are pointing directly forward

>> **advice** for beginners

When you start any new exercise program, it can be exhilarating and daunting at the same time. You obviously want to have fun as you progress through your dance workouts, but you also need to know how to work effectively and safely so that you will avoid injury.

Important points to think about before you begin to exercise are what clothing and equipment you will require; the space you will need; staying hydrated; correct breathing as you exercise; how frequently you should exercise; and how to practice safely. As a beginner to dance, you may also want to know a little about how dancers count the music.

Clothing and equipment

Proper exercise attire will not only make you feel more comfortable while you are exercising, but can also prevent injury. Make sure your sneakers have

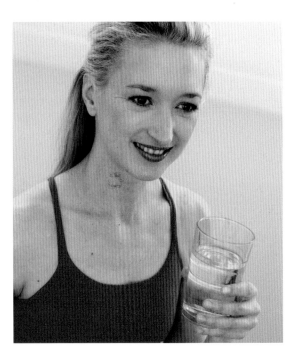

a sturdy sole and offer proper support around your ankle. Clothing should be comfortable and form-fitting, and should be made out of a material that allows the skin to breathe. You want to avoid lots of zippers, buttons, or flowing material. Zippers and buttons can scratch, and excess material will get in the way while you are moving. The only equipment you might need for these exercise programs is a comfortable, soft mat for the short, floor-based toning and stretching sections that end each workout. If you do not have a mat, you can use a folded blanket on the floor instead.

How much space do I need?

You will need to clear a small space in front of your television, computer, or DVD player so that you can follow along with the DVD. The space should be big enough to walk comfortably four steps forward and back, and four steps side to side. Please make sure that there are no obstacles in the way that you could trip over or bump into as you are practicing.

The importance of staying hydrated

Staying hydrated while exercising is more important than most people realize. Whenever you are performing an aerobic activity that raises the body temperature over a sustained period of time, your body naturally sweats to cool itself down. Drinking

In order to avoid the effects of dehydration, such as headaches and cramping, take small sips of water before, during, and after exercising.

Correct breathing maximizes the oxygen available. When you breathe out, feel the rib cage relax (inset); when you breathe in, feel it expand upward and sideways.

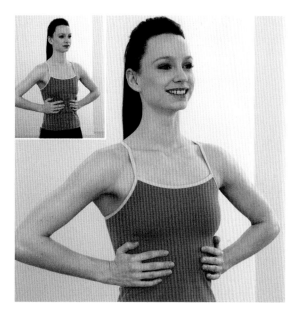

small amounts of water while you are exercising will replenish the fluid you lose through sweating. So before you start, make sure you have a glass of water conveniently placed nearby.

Correct breathing

Breathing properly during aerobic activity ensures that the lungs and heart get enough oxygen to supply the rest of the body. Think of breathing deeply and fully all the time and practice by placing your hands on the sides of your rib cage. As you inhale, slowly feel the ribs expand to the front, sides, and back. As you exhale, feel the rib cage soften as the muscles relax and the air is expelled.

How often and when should I perform these workouts?

Since these workouts last only around 15 minutes, they should easily fit into anyone's day. They can be performed at the beginning, middle, or end of your day, although I recommend exercising in the morning. This not only gets it out of the way, but you feel great for the rest of the day, too.

Try to do one of the workouts at least three times a week. Make a firm commitment to yourself to set aside regular time just for your dance. Once you get into the habit, you will feel better, more energized, and toned for everything else you do.

Counting the eights

Counting music is easy. Music is divided into regular, rhythmic beats grouped in phrases. All the music for these workouts is written in eight-count phrases. When you first perform a movement, you will repeat it for four eight-count phrases, which gives you a chance to get used to doing it. As you start to come down the aerobic curve (see p14), you only repeat the movements for two eight-count phrases. But if you ever have trouble finding the beat of the music, don't worry: All you need to do is follow along with the DVD.

>> **some safety** guidelines

Exercising safely is key. Proper alignment and technique will help keep you fit and healthy as your program becomes more advanced and in the years to come.

- **Whether your knees are bent or straight,** make sure they are always in a direct line with your toes. If the line of the knee is on the inside or outside of the foot, it places unnecessary strain on the knee joint.

- **Keep your knees soft.** Landing on a stiff leg can not only jar the body, but can also damage the joints.

- **When you jump,** think of rolling through the feet, starting from the toes, then the arches, and finally the heels.

- **Always think** of pulling your tummy in and lengthening your tailbone down toward the ground. This stops you from arching your back, which puts too much strain on the muscles supporting your spine and can damage the spinal column.

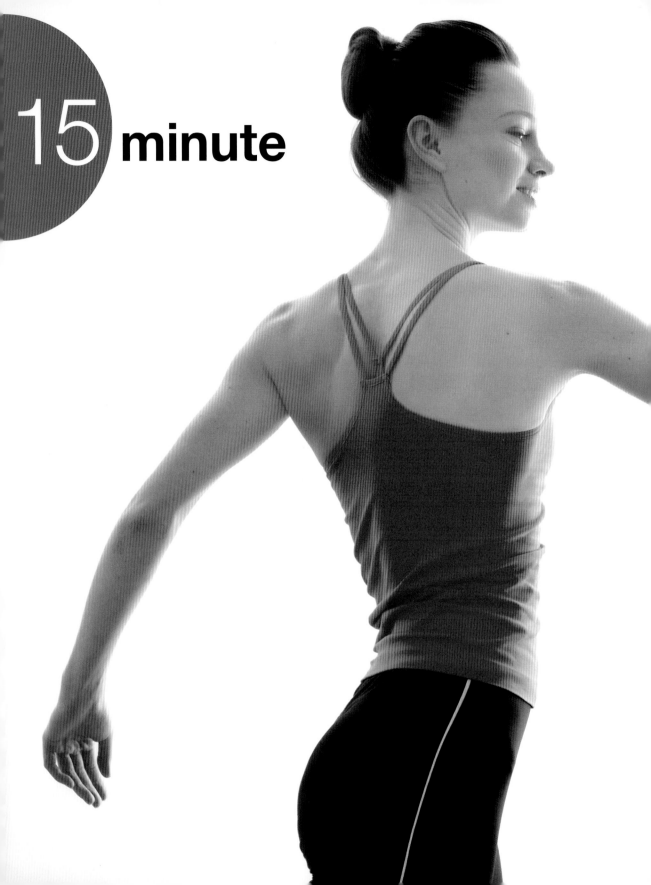

15 minute

salsa
workout >>

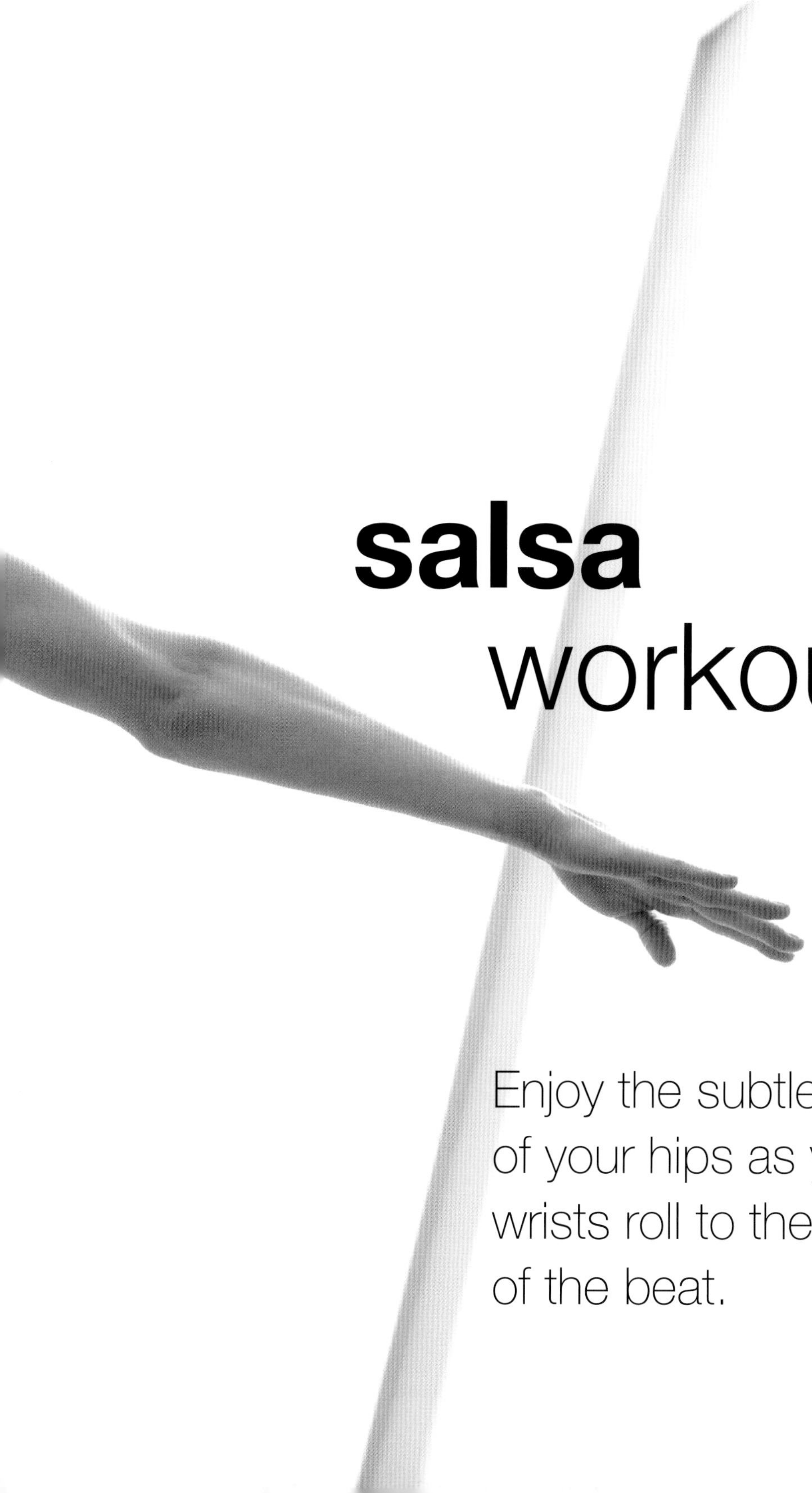

Enjoy the subtle swing
of your hips as your
wrists roll to the rhythm
of the beat.

1 **Shoulder circles** Start with your feet hip-width apart and parallel. Bend your knees. As you straighten them, start circling your shoulders forward. As you bend your knees again, you should be finishing the shoulder circle. Circle 4 times forward, then 4 times back.

2 **Head looks** Straighten your knees and lengthen through the top of your head toward the ceiling. Look over your right shoulder. Bring your head back to center, then look over your left shoulder. Repeat, alternating sides for 4 reps (1 rep = both sides).

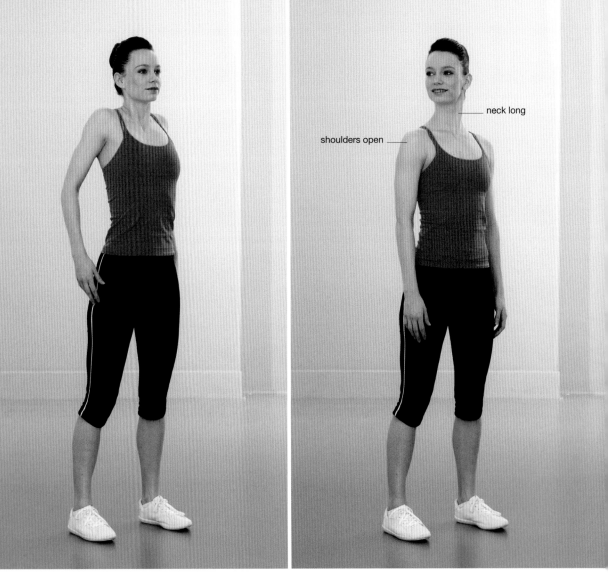

neck long

shoulders open

3 **Hip & hand circles** Start with your feet hip-width apart and softly bend your knees. Keeping your torso still and your arms straight, circle your hips and wrists. Circle 4 times to the left and 4 times to the right.

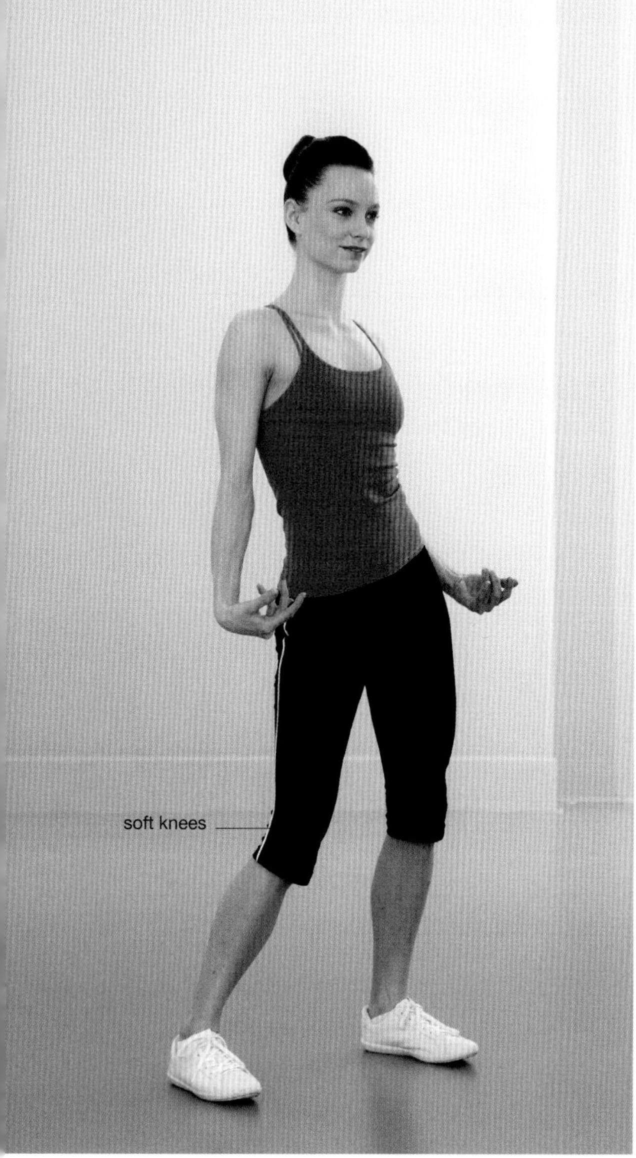

4 **Side stretch** Keeping your knees bent, place your left hand on your hip and your right arm straight beside your ear. Reach out of your hip socket and lengthen your torso to the left, stretching out the right side of your body. Slowly come back to center and repeat to the other side.

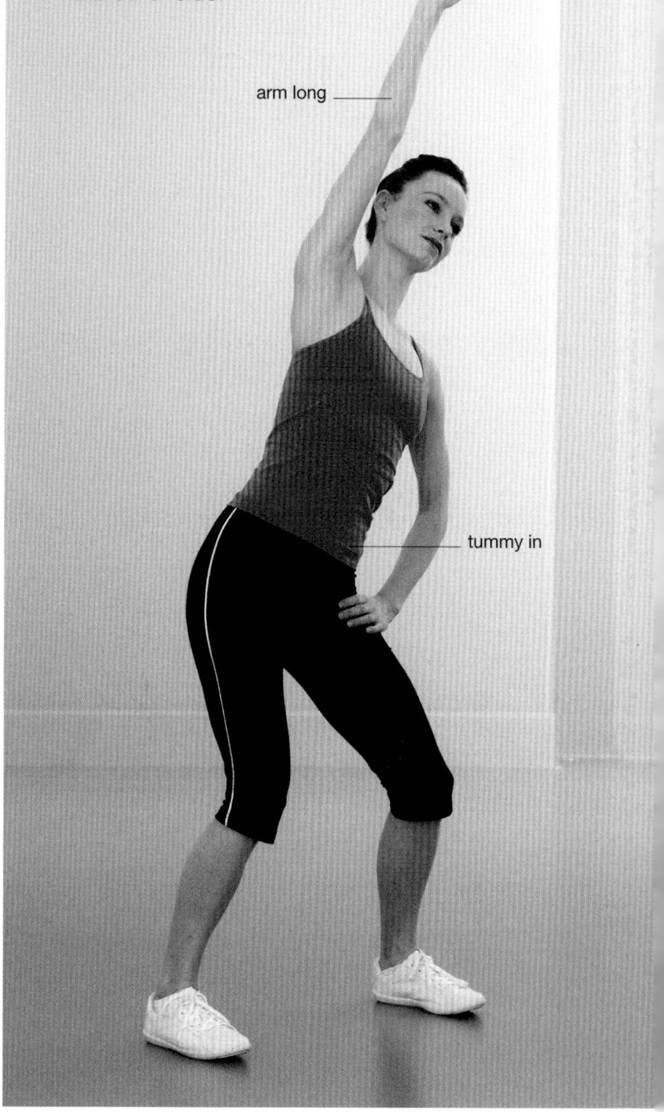

arm long

tummy in

soft knees

>> **aerobic** salsa 1

5 **Salsa 1** Place your hands on your hips with your feet together. Take a small step forward with your right foot and let your right hip swing slightly sideways. Bring your right foot back underneath you. Repeat, taking a small step forward with your left foot, then bringing it back.

6 Then take a small step back with your right foot, again letting your hip swing to the right. Bring it back underneath you. Repeat back with the left. Repeat Steps 5 and 6 one more time.

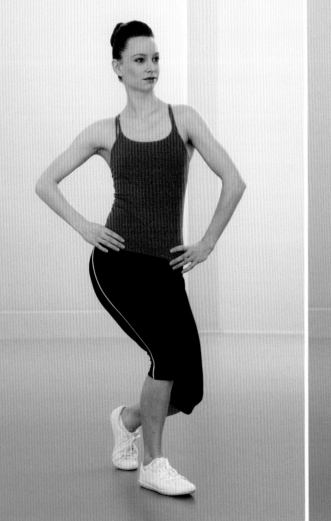

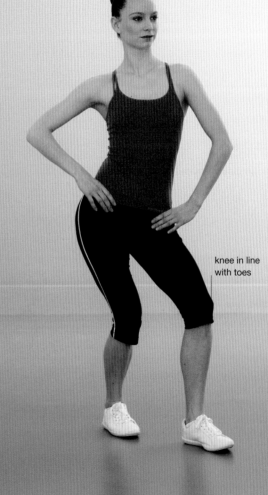

knee in line
with toes

7 **Cross forward 1** Keep your hands on your hips and cross your left foot in front of your right, bringing your right shoulder forward slightly and letting your left hip swing out.

8 Step on your right foot as you bring your left shoulder slightly forward and your right hip swings out. Bring your right foot back to center. Repeat Steps 7 and 8 for a total of 4 reps, continuing to move the shoulders in opposition to the feet.

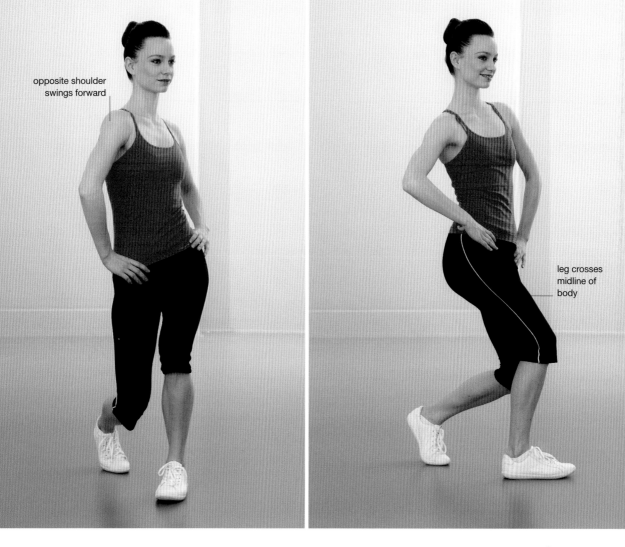

opposite shoulder swings forward

leg crosses midline of body

9 **Mambo 1** Keep your hands on your hips and cross your left foot in front of your right. Keep your left leg straight and rock onto your toes long enough to lift your right foot off the floor and place it back down underneath you.

10 Reach your left leg straight out behind you and slightly out to the left. Rock up onto your toes long enough to lift your right foot off the floor and place it back down. Repeat with your left foot crossing in front and rocking onto it. Then step your left foot next to your right, making three tiny steps underneath you, getting ready to repeat to the other side. Repeat Steps 9 and 10 for 2 reps.

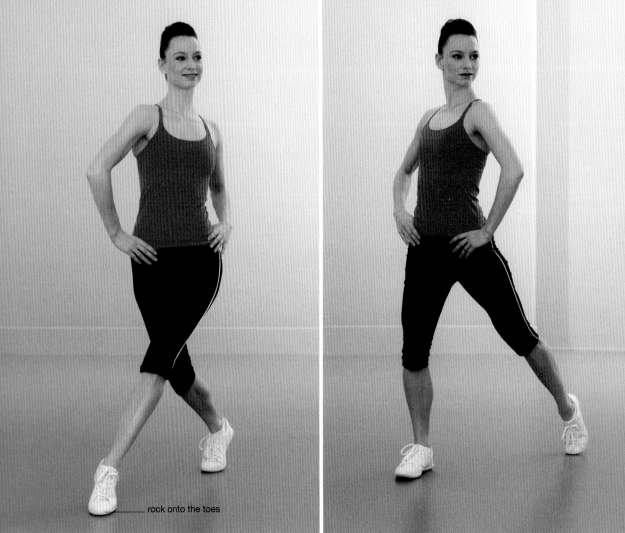

rock onto the toes

11 **Double side step 1** Place your hands on your hips and step sideways with your right foot. Step your left foot in to meet the right, and then step sideways with your right foot again. Bring your left foot in again to meet the right, this time touching the toes to the floor next to your right foot.

12 Repeat, starting with the left foot stepping to the left side. Let the hips rise and fall with the movement of the feet. Repeat Steps 11 and 12 for a total of 4 reps.

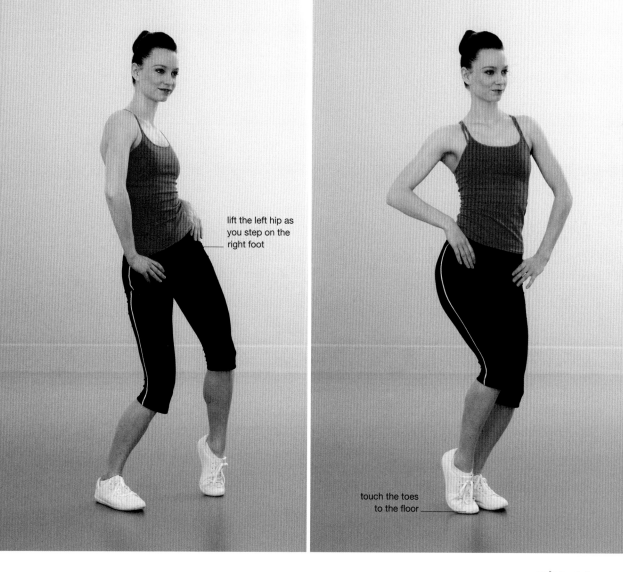

lift the left hip as you step on the right foot

touch the toes to the floor

>> **aerobic** side lunge 1

13 **Side lunge 1** Start with your hands on your hips and your feet together. Step your right leg sideways and rock up onto your toes as your right shoulder comes forward. Lift your left foot up off the floor, then place it back down.

14 Bring your right leg back underneath and repeat on the other side. Repeat Steps 13 and 14 for 4 reps.

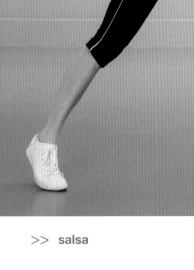

hips stay square

15 **Salsa 2** Repeat Salsa 1 (Steps 5, inset, and 6) twice, then start to raise your arms slowly to the side, making a circle with your wrists as the right leg steps forward and back. Continue raising your arms and circling your wrists as you step the left leg forward and back. Your arms should be high and your wrists circling as the right leg steps back and in, and they should be overhead as the left leg steps back. Drop your arms by your side as you step the left leg in. Repeat.

keep shoulders down

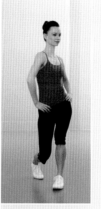

16 **Cross forward 2** Repeat Cross forward 1 (Steps 7, inset, and 8) for 4 reps, then add your arm by raising the opposite hand in line with the belly button. Make a small circle in front of you with your wrist as you cross the foot and step on it. Do a total of 4 reps.

small wrist circle

17 **Mambo 2** Repeat Mambo 1 (Steps 9, inset, and 10) for 2 reps, then, as you rock your left leg forward, circle your right arm around your head. As you rock your left leg back, make a circle down and into your body with your right arm. As you bring your left leg forward again, reach your right arm out in front. On the three quick steps, take both arms in to hip height. Repeat to the other side (shown here), then do 1 more rep.

soft hand

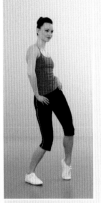

18 **Double side step 2** Repeat Double side step 1 (Steps 11, inset, and 12) for 4 reps, then bring your arms down. On the next rep, as you go to the right, bring your left leg in and skim your body with your right arm, making a circle over your head. Repeat to the other side (shown here), alternating sides for 4 reps.

tummy in

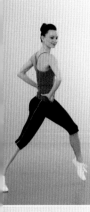

19 **Side lunge 2** Repeat Side lunge 1 (Steps 13, inset, and 14) for 4 reps, then bring your arms down. Repeat the Side lunge, but, as you rock up onto your toes on the right, bring your right arm across your body so your elbow is parallel to the floor and your hand is by your face. Make a small circle with your wrist and hand. Bring your arm down as your foot comes back to center. Repeat to the other side (shown here), alternating sides for 4 reps.

frame the face with the arm ———

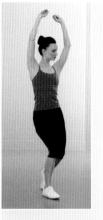

20 **Salsa 3** Repeat Salsa 2 (Step 15, inset) twice, then, on the 3rd repeat, as you step the right leg forward, bend your left arm by your left ear and make a small circle with your wrist. Bring your right leg back underneath you and your arm down and make a small jump. Repeat with the left leg forward and the right arm, and then repeat to the back. Repeat Salsa 3 one more time.

——— swing the hip

21 Cross forward 3
Repeat Cross forward 2 (Step 16, inset) for 4 reps. On the 5th rep, after you have taken the left leg forward and circled at the navel with the right hand, bring the left leg back underneath you and make a small jump before repeating to the other side. Do 4 reps of Cross forward 3.

point the toes

22 Mambo 3
Repeat Mambo 2 (Step 17, inset) for 2 reps. On the 3rd rep, instead of doing three quick steps underneath you, do a small jump. Do 2 reps of Mambo 3.

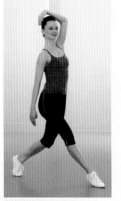

shoulders down

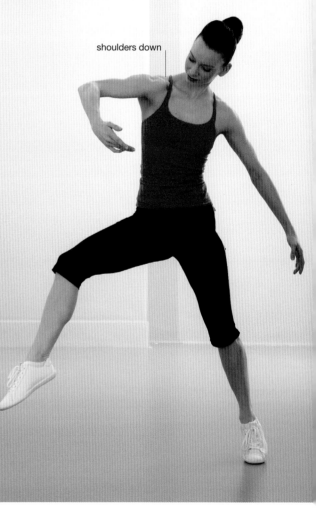

23 Double side step 3
Repeat Double side step 2 (Step 18, inset) for 4 reps, then, on the 5th rep, step on the right foot, bend the knee, lift the left foot and jump sideways, replacing the right foot with the left. Immediately step sideways again with the right foot. As you bring the left foot in to touch the right, skim the right arm over your head and back down in a graceful circle. Do 4 reps of Double side step 3.

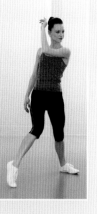

24 Side lunge 3
Repeat Side lunge 2 (Step 19, inset) for 4 reps, then bend both knees and do a small jump. As you land, bring your right leg out and your right arm across your body so your wrist and hand can make a small circle by your face. Bring your arm down as you jump both feet together again. Do 8 reps of Side lunge 3.

Now repeat all the Level 3 steps, then repeat them again in reverse order. You have reached the height of your aerobic curve. Finally, repeat the entire sequence in reverse order, starting with Step 24, working back to Step 5, and cutting the number of reps in half to bring your heart rate slowly back to rest.

back long

knee over toes

>> **tone & stretch** abs/hamstrings

25 **Abs** Lie on your back with your hands laced behind your head, knees bent, and feet together. Extend your right leg, keeping your knees together. Inhale to prepare. As you exhale, lift your head up off the floor using your abdominal muscles and your arms (inset). Do 8 reps. Inhale to prepare for the next rep, but this time, as you exhale, twist your upper torso and bend your right knee into your chest, moving your left elbow toward your right knee. Do 8 reps, then repeat to the other side, starting with your left leg straight.

26 **Hamstrings** Lie on your back, arms by your sides and knees bent, hip-width apart. Lengthen your right leg toward the ceiling and hold on to that leg comfortably with both hands. Breathing deeply, slowly bring your leg toward your chest, feeling a gentle stretch in the back of the raised leg. Repeat on the other side.

shoulders down

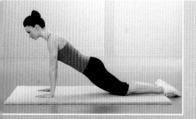

27 **Push-ups** Roll onto your knees and place your hands on the floor underneath your shoulders. Bring your knees back so that your shoulders, hips, and knees all form one straight line (inset). Inhale as you bend your elbows back to touch the sides of your rib cage. Exhale as you straighten your arms. Repeat 8 times, keeping your body in one straight line.

lengthen through
the lower back

28 **Hip stretch** Bring your right leg forward between your hands, keeping your left knee behind you. Gently press your hips forward toward your right heel. If you can, take both hands off the floor and place them on top of your right knee. Keep your back long as you breathe into your hip stretch. Repeat to the other side.

knee in line
with foot

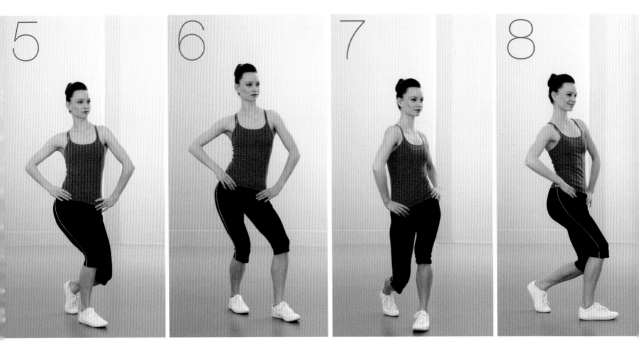

▲ **Aerobic** Salsa 1, page 22

▲ **Aerobic** Salsa 1, page 22

▲ **Aerobic** Cross forward 1, page 23

▲ **Aerobic** Cross forward 1, page 23

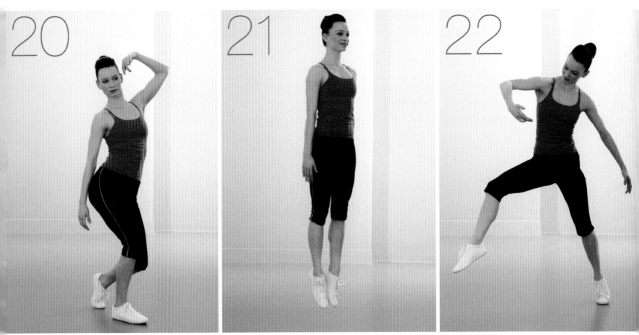

▲ **Aerobic** Salsa 3, page 29

▲ **Aerobic** Cross forward 3, page 30

▲ **Aerobic** Mambo 3, page 30

salsa at a glance

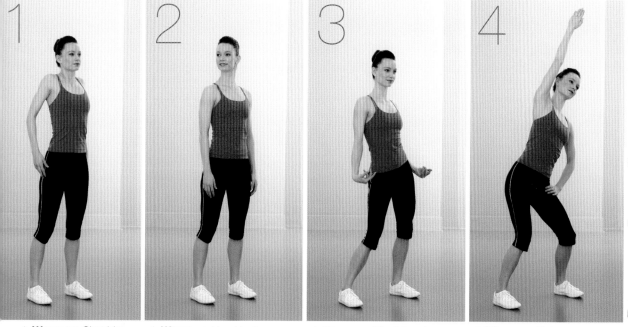

▲ **Warm-up** Shoulder circles, page 20

▲ **Warm-up** Head looks, page 20

▲ **Warm-up** Hip & hand circles, page 21

▲ **Warm-up** Side stretch, page 21

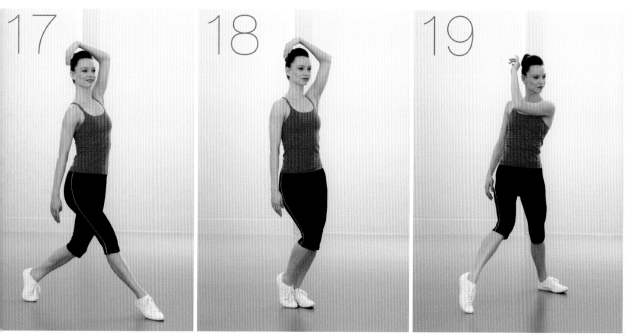

▲ **Aerobic** Mambo 2, page 28

▲ **Aerobic** Double side step 2, page 28

▲ **Aerobic** Side lunge 2, page 29

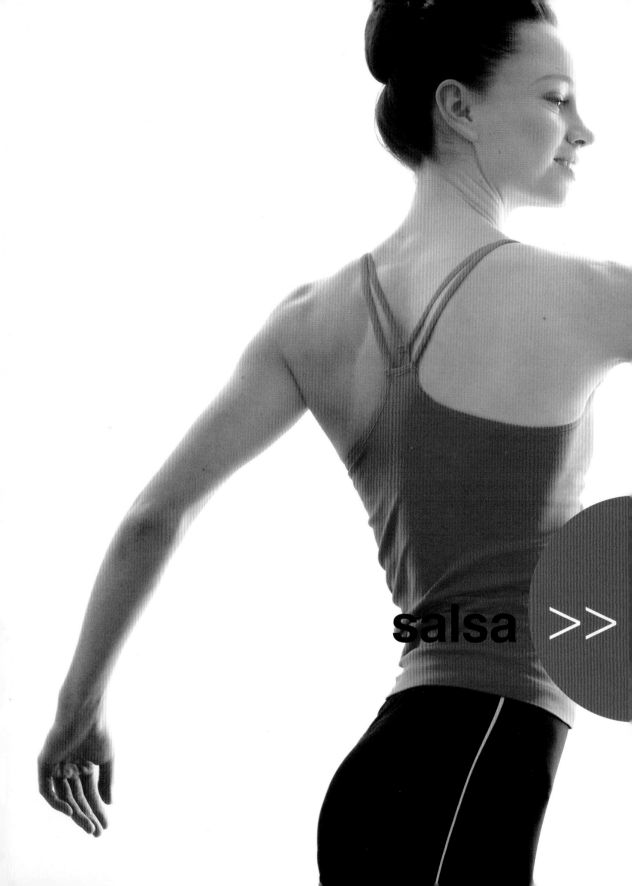

salsa >>

15 minute **summary**

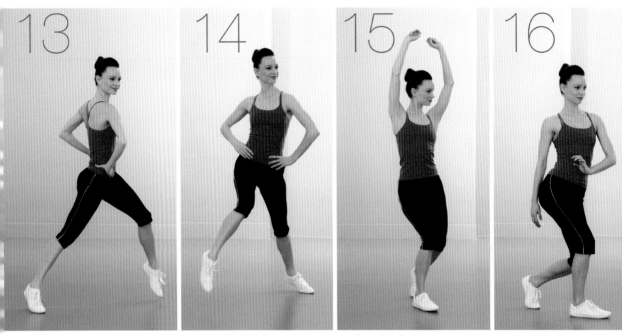

▲ **Aerobic** Side lunge 1, page 26

▲ **Aerobic** Side lunge 1, page 26

▲ **Aerobic** Salsa 2, page 27

▲ **Aerobic** Cross forward 2, page 27

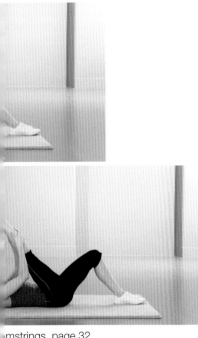

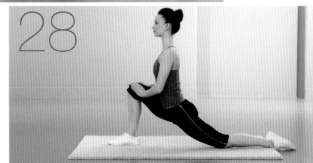

▲ **Tone & stretch** Push-ups, page 33

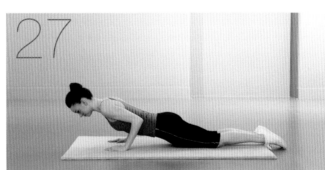

mstrings, page 32

▲ **Tone & stretch** Hip stretch, page 33

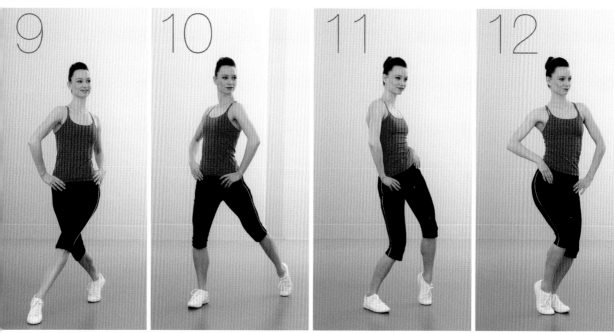

▲ **Aerobic** Mambo 1, page 24

▲ **Aerobic** Mambo 1, page 24

▲ **Aerobic** Double side step 1, page 25

▲ **Aerobic** Double side step 1, page 25

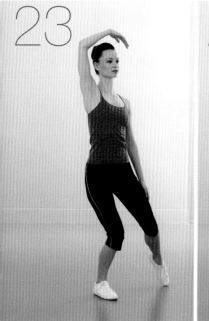

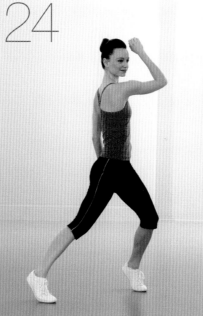

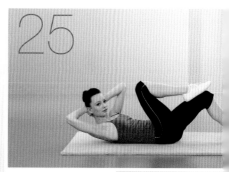

▲ **Tone & stretch** Abs, page 32

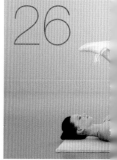

▲ **Aerobic** Double side step 3, page 31

▲ **Aerobic** Side lunge 3, page 31

▲ **Tone & stretch** H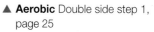

>> **salsa** FAQs

The Salsa workout combines the fun, flirtatious aspects of salsa dancing with great aerobic endurance. Here are a few extra tips and guidelines to help you understand not only the mechanics behind the steps, but also why you are doing each step.

 ### Why do I need to warm up?

Warming up the body loosens the joints and releases energy, creating heat. When the muscles and joints are warm, they function more efficiently and effectively. If your muscles and joints are supple and warm, you are less likely to get injured. This prepares your body for more vigorous exercise.

 ### How wide should I step on Salsa 1, 2, and 3?

Remember, salsa is really a couple's dance, so if you were to take very large steps, you would step on your partner's feet. Practice as though you were in a salsa club, with small steps forward and back for the salsa, and small steps sideways for the Double side step.

>> ### Whenever I'm circling my arm overhead, I don't feel very sensuous.

The circle of the arm around the head and down is not meant to feel like brushing away a fly! The arm movement draws attention to the space between your arm and the line of your body. It is expressive and alluring without actually touching your skin. A good way to practice this is to stand in front of the mirror and run your hands over your body about an inch (2.5cm) away. Can you see your arm following the contour of your body? That is exactly what you want to do in Mambo and Double side step.

>> ## I'm finding the movement of the hips difficult on the Double side step.

A useful tip is to imagine that you are standing between two walls. Your whole body can only move from side to side, not forward and backward. Start by working on your feet, moving side together, side together. As you step sideways, lift your opposite hip up slightly. As your feet come together, switch the hip you are lifting. This might feel awkward at first, but the more you practice, the better you will get.

>> ## Can you explain the small circle with the wrist on Side lunge?

The nature of salsa is very subtle. You want to relax your hand as much as possible. Think of your wrist making a small, delicate circle inward. Once you have the action of the wrist, you can place it anywhere near your body in a graceful, caressing movement.

>> ## What is the difference between doing an aerobic workout and toning and stretching?

Aerobic exercise strengthens the heart and lungs. Toning builds muscular strength, while stretching lengthens the muscles. For total fitness, you want to work on each equally. Problems arise when people work really hard on one aspect of training, and ignore the others. For example, people who concentrate all their efforts on strengthening their muscles and never stretch them will build short, tight muscles that have a limited range of motion.

Shifting the weight onto the toes in the Mambo step is quite difficult. How do I do it?

When we are walking, we don't even think about shifting the weight of the body from one foot to the other, so the Mambo step is less difficult than you might think. You want to shift your weight just enough to lift your other foot off the floor and place it back down, without actually transferring the weight from the foot that is underneath you.

15 minute

Soft arms.
Graceful feet.
Poise. Elegance.
The beauty
of the ballet.

ballet
workout >>

>> **warm-up** prances/port de bras

1 **Prances** Start with your toes apart, heels together. Relax your arms by your sides with your fingertips curving softly toward each other. Lift your heels off the floor. Bend your right knee as your left heel comes back into the starting position. This stretches your ankles and toes. Repeat, alternating sides for 4 reps (1 rep = both sides).

2 **Port de bras** On the 5th rep, bring your arms forward, above your head, to the side, and down. Then reverse, taking your arms to the side, above your head, forward, and down.

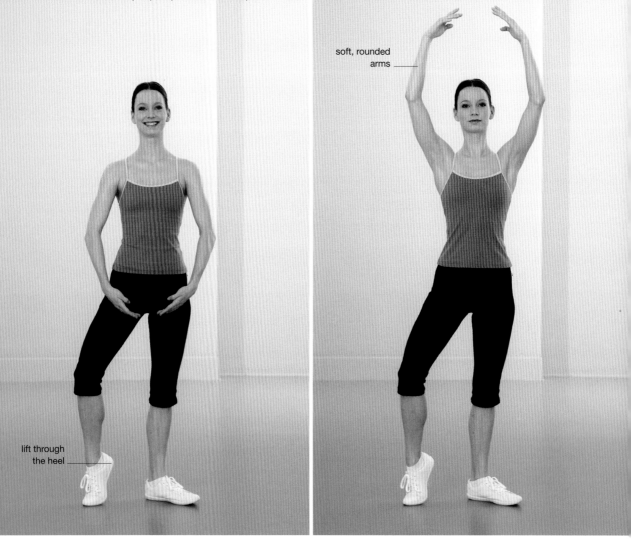

soft, rounded arms _____

lift through the heel _____

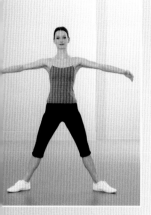

3 2nd position plié

Place the feet just beyond shoulder width, toes slightly turned out from the hip socket. Slowly raise the arms to shoulder height, with the palms facing forward and the fingers long (inset). Bend the knees over the toes as the arms swing down and cross in front of you at the wrists. As you straighten the legs, swing the arms back up to shoulder height. Do a total of 4 reps.

4 Side lunge

Bend your right knee while keeping your left leg straight and your hips square. Lengthen your left arm over your head as you stretch out the left side of your body. Straighten your right knee as you bring your arms back to your side. Repeat Step 3, then Step 4, stretching to the other side.

one long, straight line from shoulder, to hip, to foot

knees over toes

>> **aerobic** hamstring curls 1

5 **Hamstring curls 1** Place your hands on your hips as you step on your right foot. Bend your left knee behind you so that your left foot lengthens toward your bottom. Keep your navel pulled into your spine so that your back stays lengthened. Place your left foot back onto the floor, feet hip-width apart and knees soft.

6 Repeat to the other side, then repeat Steps 5 and 6, alternating sides for 8 reps. This will help to warm up your body and mobilize your joints.

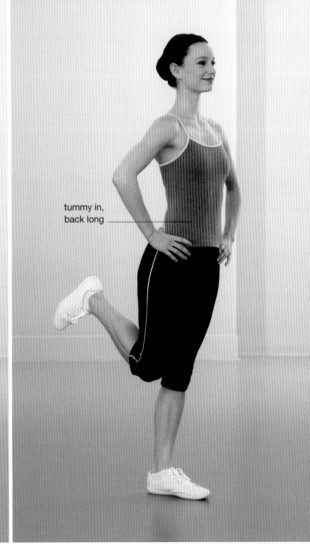

tummy in,
back long

7 **Forward & back 1** Relax your arms by your sides and walk forward, starting on your right foot. Walk three steps forward and then bring your left foot to touch next to your right.

8 Then walk three steps backward and bring your right foot to touch next to your left. Keep your shoulders open and your head lengthening toward the ceiling. Repeat Steps 7 and 8 for a total of 4 reps.

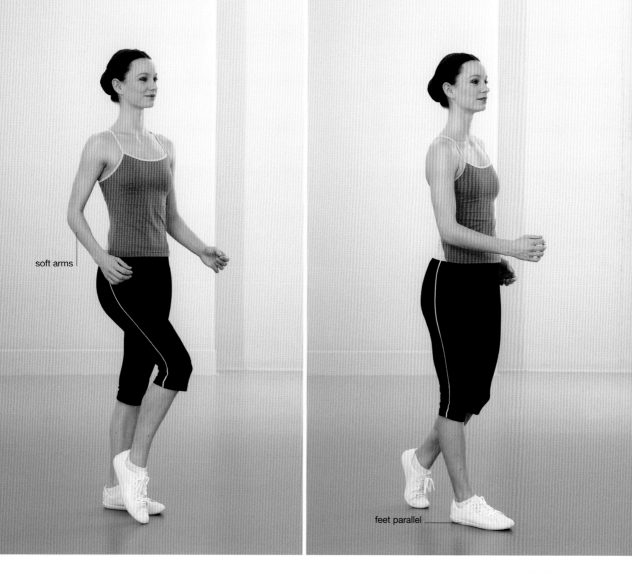

soft arms

feet parallel

>> **aerobic** attitude 1

9 **Attitude 1** Place your hands on your hips as you step onto your right foot. Bend your left leg, lifting your knee to hip height. Pull your tummy in. Keep your shoulders and hips square.

10 Place your left foot back onto the floor, feet hip-width apart and knees soft, then lift your right knee to hip height. Repeat Steps 9 and 10, alternating sides for 8 reps.

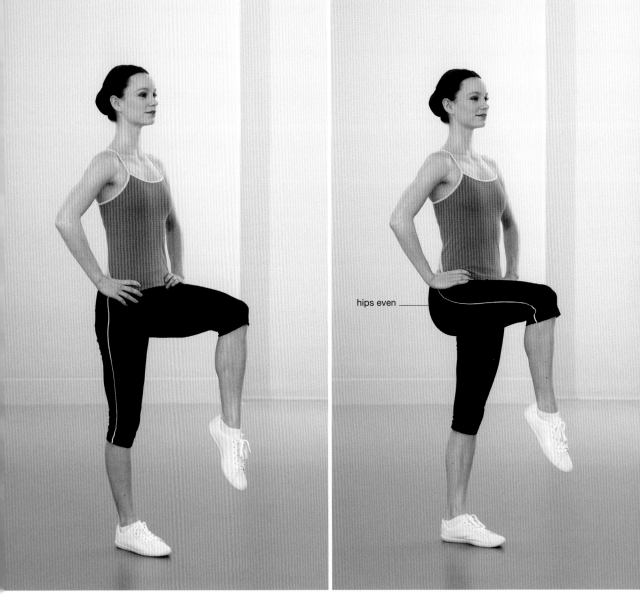

hips even

11 **Passé 1** Slightly turn out your feet from the hip sockets and relax your arms by your sides with your elbows lifted. Softly curve your fingertips. Step on your right foot and bend your left knee, touching the toes of your left foot to your right knee. Your left leg should be slightly turned out so that your hip, knee, and foot are all in one straight line.

12 Place your left foot on the floor so that your feet are shoulder-width apart, then repeat, lifting your right foot off the floor. Repeat Steps 11 and 12, alternating sides for a total of 8 reps.

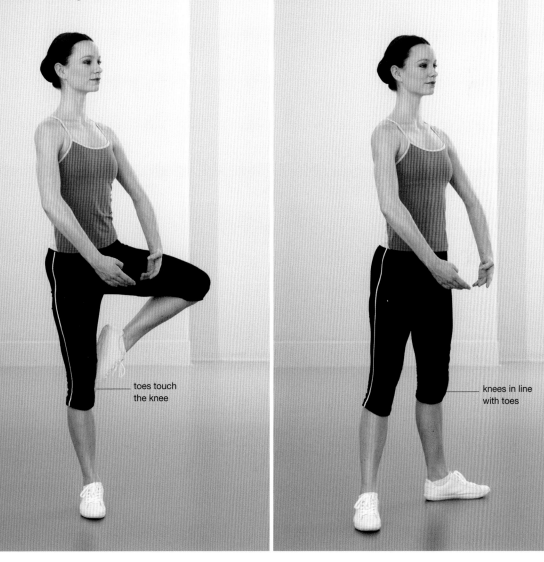

toes touch
the knee

knees in line
with toes

>> **aerobic** toe taps 1

13 **Toe taps 1** Start with your feet slightly turned out from your hip sockets, your arms relaxed and your fingertips rounded. Step on your right foot and point your left foot, tapping your toes lightly on the floor.

14 Bend your knees as you transfer your weight onto your left foot, then straighten your legs as you tap the toes of your right foot on the floor. Repeat Steps 13 and 14, alternating sides for a total of 8 reps. Make sure your feet and knees are in proper alignment throughout.

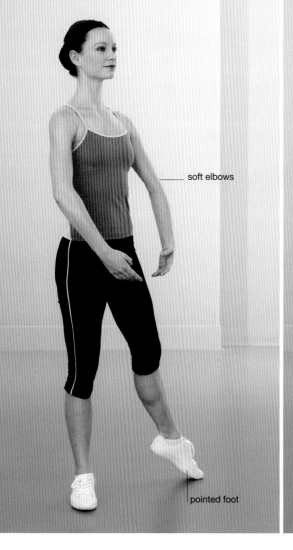

soft elbows

pointed foot

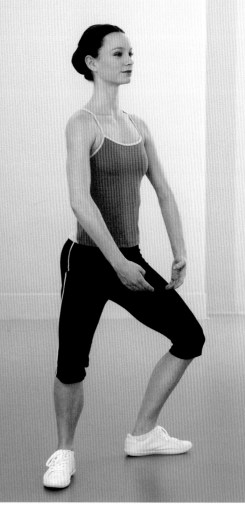

15 **Hamstring curls 2** Repeat Hamstring curls 1 (Steps 5, inset, and 6) for 8 reps, then bend your knees, step on your right foot, and swing both arms toward your hips. As your left knee bends behind you, swing your left arm to the left and your right arm in front of you. Repeat to the other side (shown here), then alternate sides for a total of 8 reps.

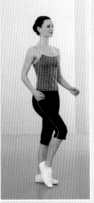

16 **Forward & back 2** Repeat Forward & back 1 (Steps 7, inset, and 8) for 4 reps, then, on the 5th rep, as you walk forward, circle your arms forward, overhead, then sideways. As you touch the left foot next to the right, cross your arms at the wrists in front. As you walk backward, reverse the arm circle, starting to the side. Do a total of 4 reps.

elbow soft and lifted

fingers long

long arms

knee in line with toes

>> **aerobic** attitude 2/passé 2

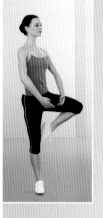

17 **Attitude 2** Repeat Attitude 1 (Steps 9, inset, and 10) for 8 reps, then step on your right foot. Take your arms up, fingers soft, then bend your left knee to hip height. Bring your right elbow toward your left knee and take your left arm gracefully out to your left side. Repeat to the other side (shown here), then alternate sides for a total of 8 reps.

18 **Passé 2** Repeat Passé 1 (Steps 11, inset, and 12) for 8 reps, then bend your right knee and transfer your weight onto your right leg, arms softly down by your sides. As you point your left foot toward your right knee and straighten your right leg, swing your right arm to the right and your left arm in front. Repeat, alternating sides for a total of 8 reps.

forearm
parallel to floor

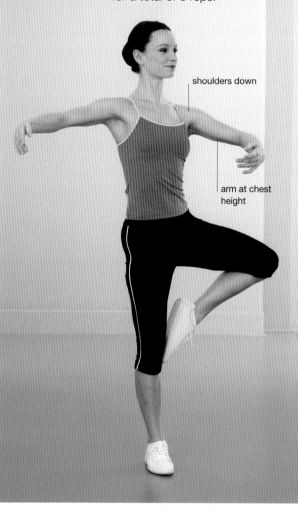

shoulders down

arm at chest
height

19 **Toe taps 2** Repeat Toe taps 1 (Steps 13, inset, and 14) for 8 reps, then twist the upper torso to the right as you step on the right foot. Point the left foot, tapping the toes on the floor as you swing the arms softly to the right. Repeat to the other side (shown here), then alternate sides for a total of 8 reps.

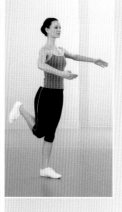

20 **Hamstring curls 3** Repeat Hamstring curls 2 (Step 15, inset) for 8 reps, then bend both knees and swing your arms to your hips. As you bend your left leg, bring your left arm forward and swing your right arm out to the side. Jump softly onto your right leg.

let the arms flow with the movement of the torso

foot pointed

Jump off the right leg and place both feet back on the floor, hip-width apart, as you swing your arms down. Repeat, alternating sides for a total of 8 reps.

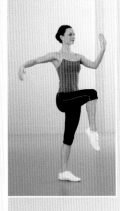

21 Forward & back 3
Repeat Forward & back 2 (Step 16, inset) for 4 reps, then take 3 steps forward, right, left, right. Then step on the left foot, step sideways on the right and, with both arms to the side, cross the left leg behind the right and stretch the left arm over your head while the right arm circles down by your hips. Then step sideways to reverse the lunge. Walk back 3 steps. Repeat.

22 Attitude 3
Repeat Attitude 2 (Step 17, inset) for 8 reps, then jump on the right foot as you bend the left knee to hip height. Bring your right elbow to your left knee, and your left arm to the side. Jump off your right foot, landing on both feet, arms overhead, to repeat to the other side. Repeat, alternating sides for a total of 8 reps.

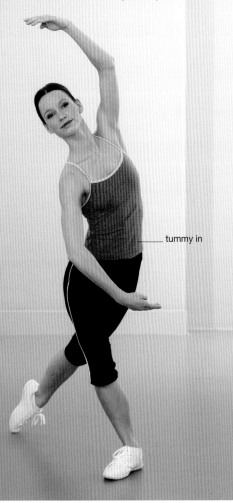

tummy in

soft arms

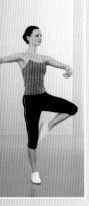

23 **Passé 3** Repeat Passé 2 (Step 18, inset) for 8 reps, then, with your legs slightly turned out, bend both knees over your toes, arms down by your sides. Jump onto your right foot, bring your left foot to touch your right knee, take your left arm in front of your chest, and your right arm out to the side. Then jump onto both feet, hip-width apart. Repeat to the other side. Repeat, alternating sides for a total of 8 reps.

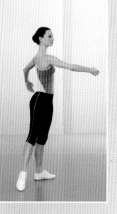

24 **Double side step jump** Repeat Toe taps 2 (Step 19, inset) for 8 reps, then step on the right foot, bend the knee, and jump sideways, replacing the right foot with the left and turning the upper torso and arms to the right. Repeat to the other side for 4 reps.

Now repeat all the Level 3 steps, then repeat them again in reverse order. You have reached the height of your aerobic curve. Finally, repeat the entire sequence in reverse order, starting with Step 24, working back to Step 5, and cutting the number of reps in half to bring your heart rate slowly back to rest.

heels together

roll through the foot to land

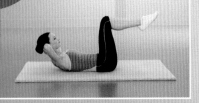

25 **Abs** Lie on your back, fingers laced behind your head. Bend both knees to your chest, then take your legs to a 90° angle. Inhale, and, as you exhale, pull your navel to your spine and slowly lift your head (inset). Inhale and relax your head down. Repeat 8 times. Next time, as you exhale, twist your upper torso, taking your left elbow toward your right knee while extending your left leg. Inhale, relax your head and leg down, then reverse. Repeat, alternating sides for a total of 4 reps.

26 **Spine** Relax your head onto the floor and hug your knees into your chest, stretching out your lower back and hip socket. Then roll your bent knees over to the right as you extend your arms sideways and turn your head to look left. Relax into the stretch before returning to center to repeat to the other side.

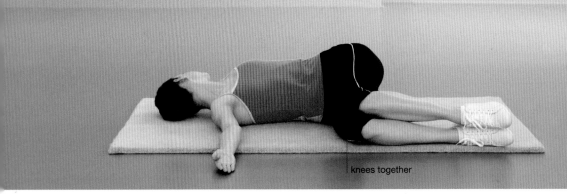

knees together

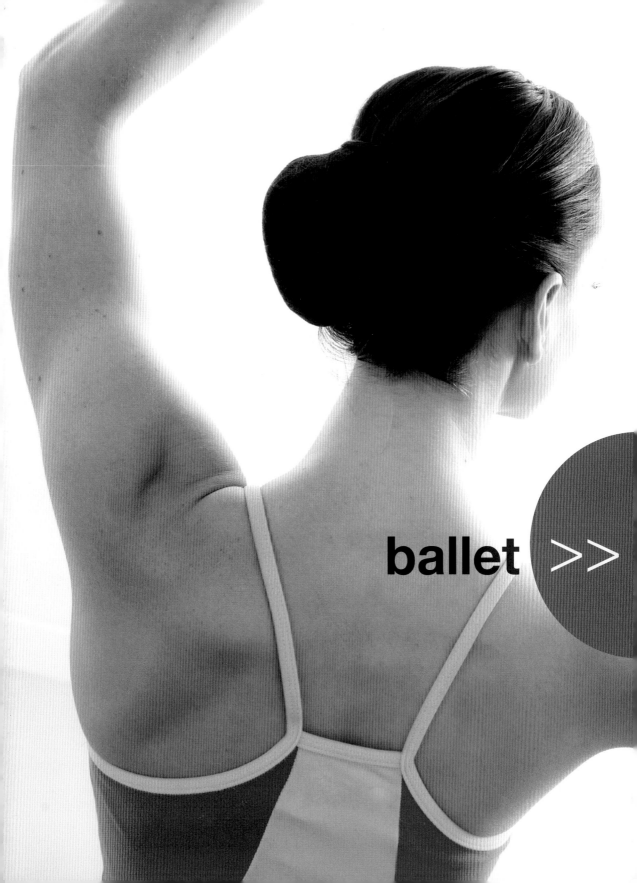

ballet >>

ballet at a glance

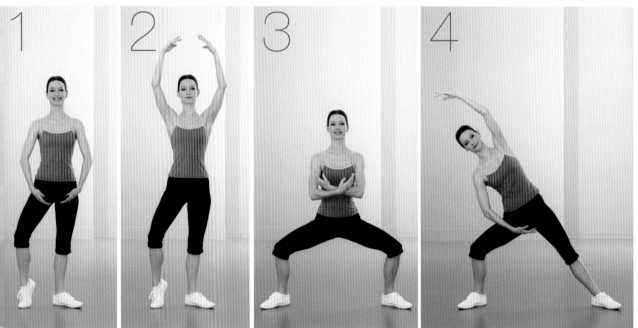

▲ **Warm-up**
Prances, page 44

▲ **Warm-up**
Port de bras, page 44

▲ **Warm-up** 2nd position plié,
page 45

▲ **Warm-up** Side lunge, page 45

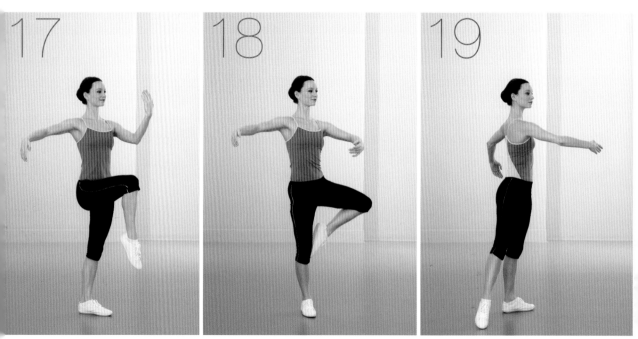

▲ **Aerobic** Attitude 2, page 52

▲ **Aerobic** Passé 2, page 52

▲ **Aerobic** Toe taps 2, page 53

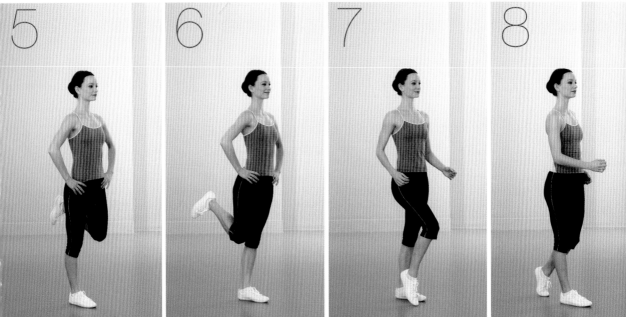

▲ **Aerobic** Hamstring curls 1, page 46

▲ **Aerobic** Hamstring curls 1, page 46

▲ **Aerobic** Forward & back 1, page 47

▲ **Aerobic** Forward & back 1, page 47

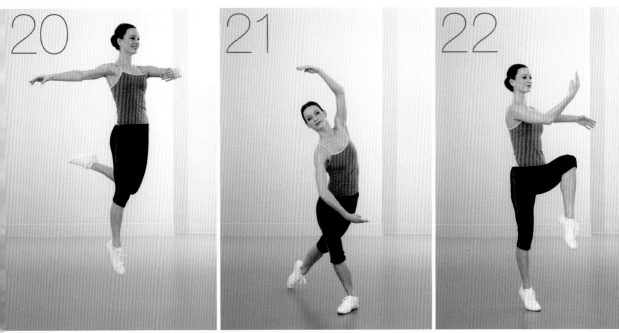

▲ **Aerobic** Hamstring curls 3, page 53

▲ **Aerobic** Forward & back 3, page 54

▲ **Aerobic** Attitude 3, page 54

27 **Hamstrings** Lie on your back with your arms down by your sides, feet on the floor and knees bent, hip-width apart. Lengthen the right leg toward the ceiling and hold onto it comfortably with both hands. Breathing deeply, slowly bring that leg toward your chest, feeling a gentle stretch in the back of the leg. Repeat on the other side.

28 **Side** Sit up tall, legs crossed. Lengthen your left arm up toward the ceiling, with your right arm down by your side, palm facing down. Slowly bend to the right, stretching out the left side of your body. Come back to center and repeat to the other side.

stretch through the side

15 minute **summary**

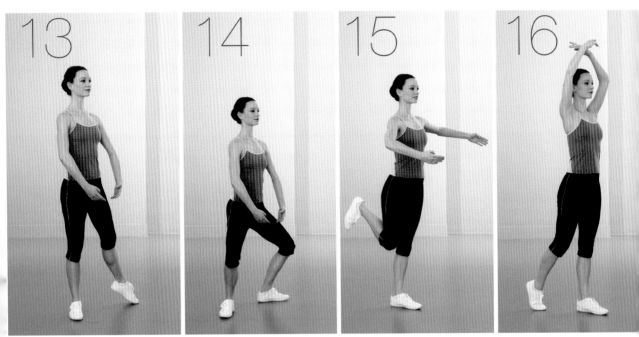

▲ **Aerobic** Toe taps 1, page 50

▲ **Aerobic** Toe taps 1, page 50

▲ **Aerobic** Hamstring curls 2, page 51

▲ **Aerobic** Forward & back 2, page 51

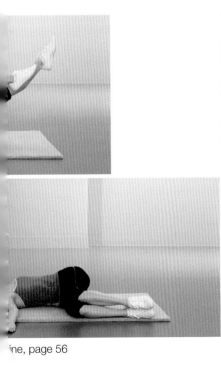

ne, page 56

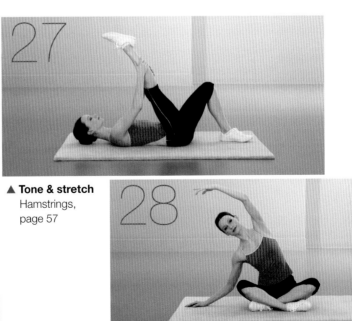

▲ **Tone & stretch** Hamstrings, page 57

▲ **Tone & stretch** Side, page 57

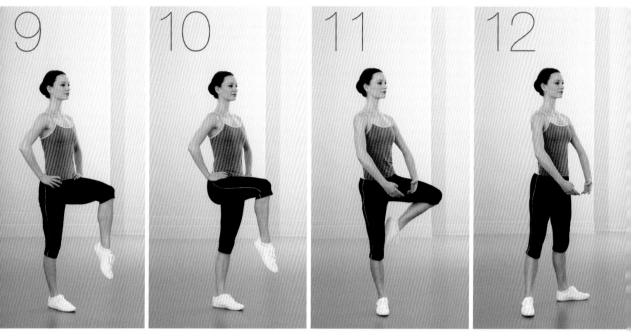

▲ **Aerobic** Attitude 1, page 48

▲ **Aerobic** Attitude 1, page 48

▲ **Aerobic** Passé 1, page 49

▲ **Aerobic** Passé 1, page 49

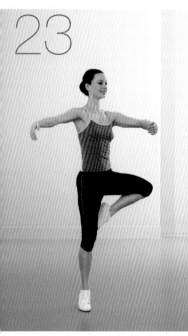

▲ **Aerobic** Passé 3, page 55

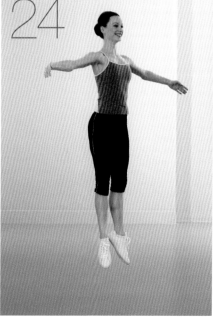

▲ **Aerobic** Double side step jump, page 55

▲ **Tone & stretch**
Abs, page 56

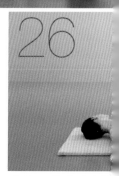

▲ **Tone & stretch** S·

>> **ballet** FAQs

The Ballet workout combines the grace and beauty of ballet with the cardiovascular endurance of aerobics. Learning to keep the poise and elegance of the balletic arms while working on strength and stamina increases coordination, muscular definition, cardiovascular fitness, endurance, and flexibility.

>> ### I've never done ballet before. How do I get my arms to look graceful?

The key to having beautiful, balletic arms is to lengthen through your fingertips. You want to think of extending through space as you move. Pretend your arms are 3 feet (1 meter) longer than they are and that you are trying to paint the walls, ceiling, and floor every time you move. The elbows should always be soft and lifted and the shoulders should be down.

>> ### How turned out should my legs be in Passé 1, 2, and 3?

Most dancers work for years on their turn-out, often forcing it, which has dire consequences for the knees. You want to rotate the leg from the hip socket, not the other way around. Try to have the legs turned out equally from the hips, in a comfortable position. The most important aspect is not the amount of turn-out you have, but that the hip, knee, and foot are all turned out evenly and point in the same direction.

>> ### Why is it important to have my knees and toes facing the same direction?

In ballet, turning out from the hips through the knees and feet is extremely important, and not just for aesthetic reasons. By keeping the alignment of your body within your range of motion, you are protecting your joints from wear and tear. If you let the knee roll inward, you would put unnecessary strain on the inner part of the knee joint. Conversely, if you let the toes roll in and the knees roll out, you would be putting strain on the outside of the knee joint.

What do the Toe taps 1, 2, and 3 do for the body?

Toe taps 1 help to mobilize the joints in the legs and feet and they warm up the body through the shifting of the weight. In Toe taps 2, the spine starts to loosen. By keeping the hips still and twisting, the chest—in other words, the upper vertebrae in the back—are stretched and rotated. In Toe taps 3, a sideways jump is added to raise the heart rate.

Do my heels need to be placed on the floor after each jump of Hamstring curls 3?

Yes. Definitely yes. When you are jumping, you should always place the whole foot on the floor after each jump. Otherwise, you are putting too much pressure on your calf muscles. In order to avoid injury, be sure to roll through your whole foot on each and every jump.

My abdominal muscles feel really weak. What can I do about it?

The abdominal muscles are extremely important since they help support the spine and internal organs. Try to do a few abdominal crunches with your hands laced behind your head every morning. Step 25 on p80 offers a good example. Even doing just 10 simple crunches will help to strengthen your stomach muscles and support your spine and back for the rest of the day.

I'm not sure of the feet on Forward & back 3. Can you please explain how the lunge works?

This movement is challenging since the feet change from being parallel when you are walking forward to being turned out to the side. The weight of your body stays on the front leg while you point your other foot to the back and circle the arms. Always be sure to have the knees over the toes, both when the feet are parallel and when they are turned out.

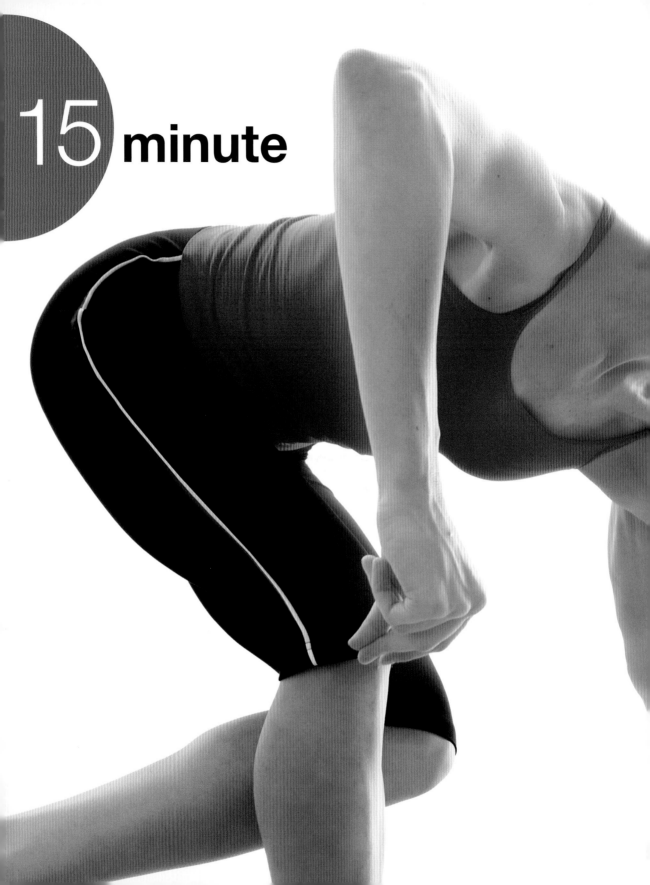

15 minute

jazz
workout >>

Snap your fingers.
Roll your shoulders.
Dance your way to
a better body.

1 **Plié shoulder circles** Start with your feet hip-width apart and parallel. Bend your knees. As you straighten them, start circling your right shoulder forward. As you bend your knees again, you should finish the shoulder circle. Repeat with your left shoulder. Repeat, alternating sides for 4 reps (1 rep = both sides), then do 4 reps circling the shoulders backward.

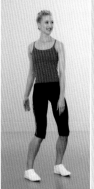

2 **Torso twist** Keep your feet hip-width apart and bend your knees. As you straighten them, twist your upper torso to the right, keeping your hips square (inset). As you bend your knees again, bring your shoulders back to center to repeat to the other side. Repeat, alternating sides for 8 reps.

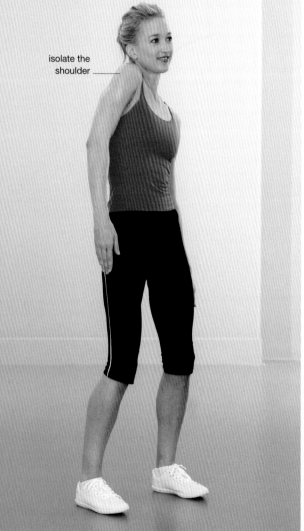

isolate the shoulder _____

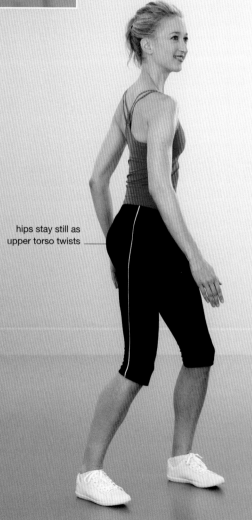

hips stay still as upper torso twists _____

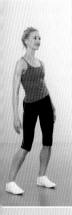

3 **Hip side to side** Relax your arms by your sides and softly bend your knees. Lift your right hip directly to the right side and let your left hip sink toward the floor. Bring your hips back to center and repeat to the other side (inset). Repeat, alternating sides, for a total of 8 reps.

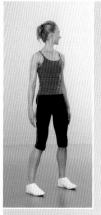

4 **Head looks** Straighten your knees and lengthen through the top of your head toward the ceiling. Look over your right shoulder. Bring your head back to center, then look over your left shoulder (inset). Repeat for 4 reps.

keep the shoulders open

don't let your hips move forward and backward as you swing side to side

>> **aerobic** ball change 1

5 **Ball change 1** Stand with your feet together and place your hands on your hips. Cross your left leg straight behind your right leg, and bring your left shoulder slightly forward. Transfer your weight onto your left foot just enough to lift up your right foot and place it back down.

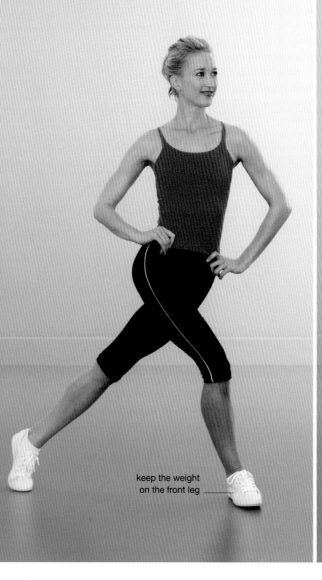

keep the weight on the front leg

6 Bring your left leg back to center and repeat to the other side. Keep your navel pulled into your spine and your back long. Repeat Steps 5 and 6 for a total of 4 reps.

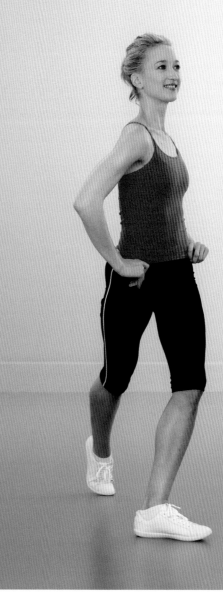

7 **Cross touch 1** Still keeping your hands on your hips, cross your left foot in front of your right foot, and step on it.

8 Bring your right foot out to the side, touch the toes of your right foot on the floor, and bring your right shoulder slightly forward. Repeat Steps 7 and 8 to the other side, then do another rep moving forward. Now do another 2 reps moving backward, then 2 more reps forward and 2 more reps backward, making a total of 8 reps.

the hips stay still as the feet move

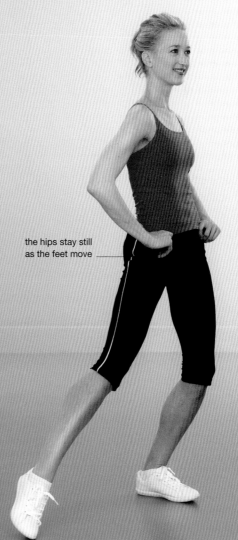

>> **aerobic** box step 1

9 **Box step 1** Place your hands on your hips and bring your feet together. Step forward on your right foot and slightly out to the right side.

10 Then step forward on your left foot and slightly to your left side. Next, step back on your right foot, bringing it back to your original starting position. Finish the Box step by bringing your left foot back next to your right. Repeat Steps 9 and 10 for a total of 8 reps. Once you have the foot pattern, try to make the opposite shoulder come slightly forward as you move each leg.

feet are parallel

11 **Grapevine 1** Relax your arms by your sides and take a small step to the side with your right foot. Lift up your left foot, cross it behind the right, and step on it.

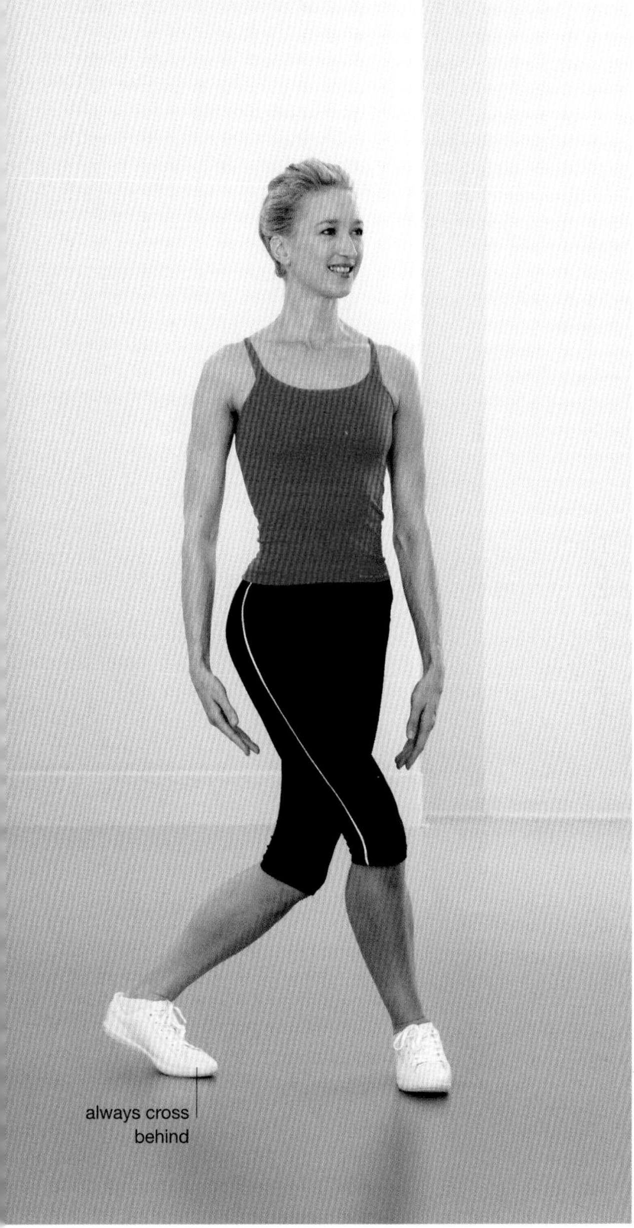

12 Lift your right foot up and again take a small step to the right side. Lift your left heel up, keeping your toes on the floor while snapping your right fingers straight down by your hips. Repeat to the left, starting with your left foot. Repeat Steps 11 and 12 for a total of 4 reps.

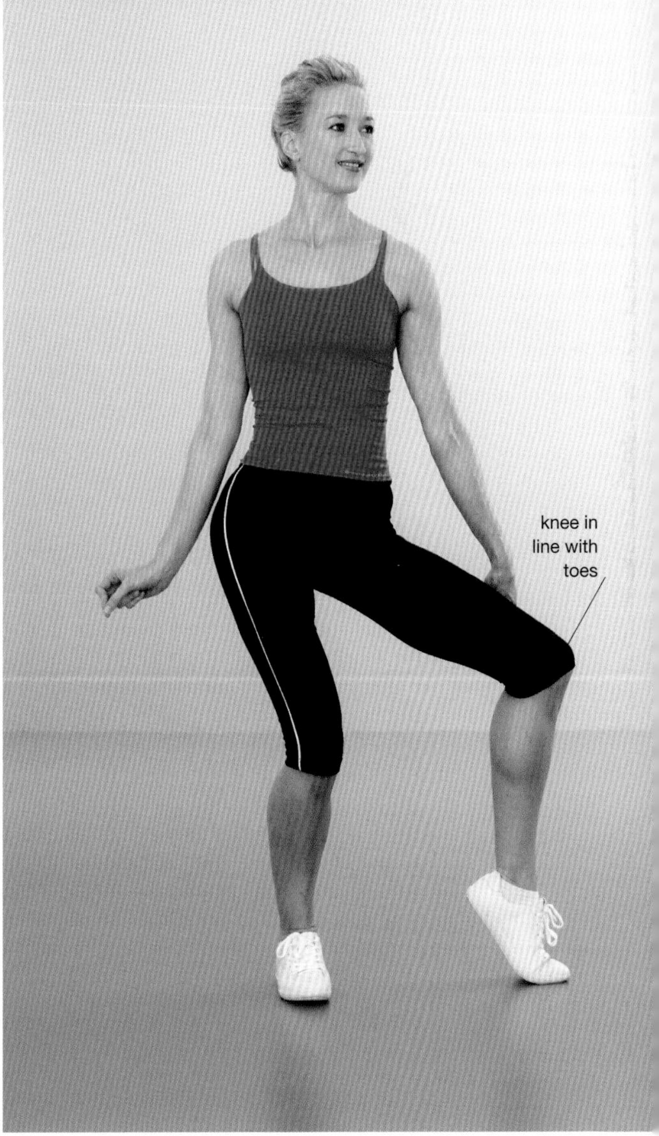

knee in
line with
toes

always cross
behind

>> **aerobic** step touch 1

13 **Step touch 1** Place your hands on your hips with your feet together. Touch the toes of your right foot out to the right side. Bring your right foot back to center.

14 Then touch the toes of your left foot out to the left side. Try to add your left shoulder coming forward as your right shoulder moves back. Repeat Steps 13 and 14 for a total of 8 reps.

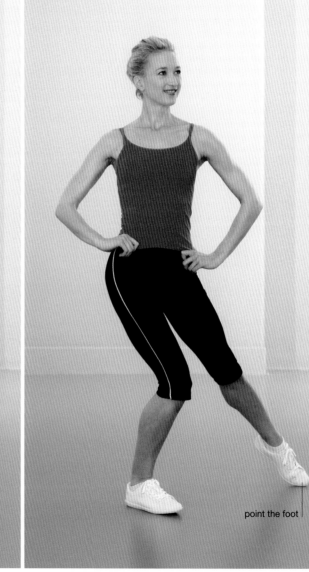

point the foot

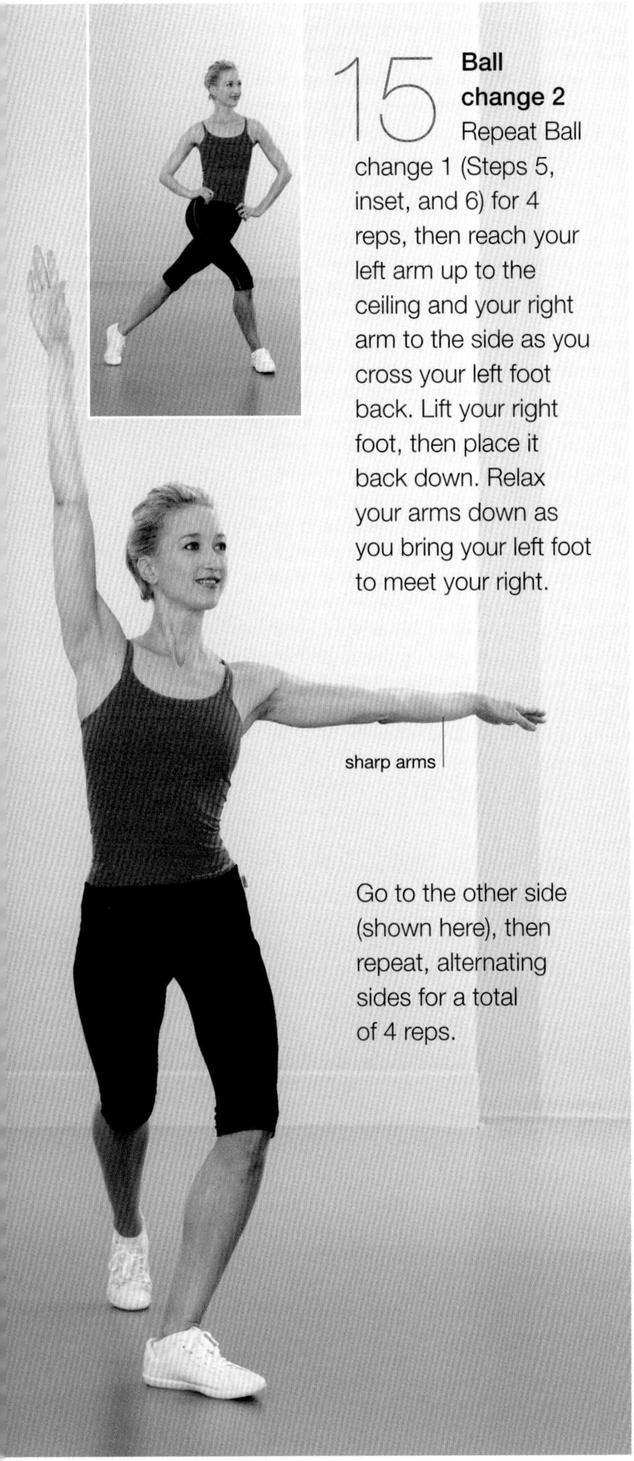

15 Ball change 2
Repeat Ball change 1 (Steps 5, inset, and 6) for 4 reps, then reach your left arm up to the ceiling and your right arm to the side as you cross your left foot back. Lift your right foot, then place it back down. Relax your arms down as you bring your left foot to meet your right.

sharp arms

Go to the other side (shown here), then repeat, alternating sides for a total of 4 reps.

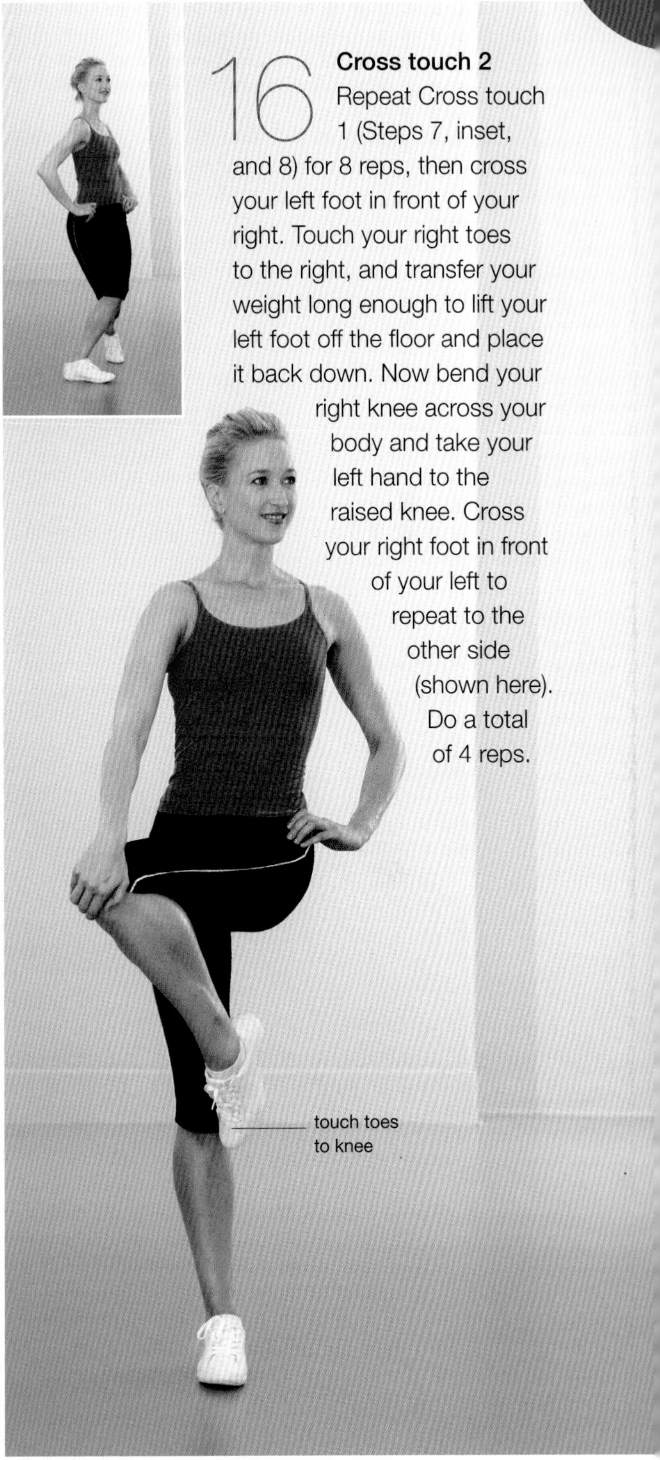

16 Cross touch 2
Repeat Cross touch 1 (Steps 7, inset, and 8) for 8 reps, then cross your left foot in front of your right. Touch your right toes to the right, and transfer your weight long enough to lift your left foot off the floor and place it back down. Now bend your right knee across your body and take your left hand to the raised knee. Cross your right foot in front of your left to repeat to the other side (shown here). Do a total of 4 reps.

touch toes to knee

>> **aerobic** box step 2/grapevine 2

17 **Box step 2** Repeat Box step 1 (Steps 9, inset, and 10) for 8 reps, then bring your left shoulder and arm forward with your hands flexed and palms facing away from you as you step forward and sideways on your right foot. Now bring your right shoulder and hand forward as you step forward and sideways on your left foot (shown here). Now step back with your right foot, then with your left, alternating feet and hands. Repeat for a total of 8 reps.

flat hands

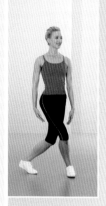

18 **Grapevine 2** Repeat Grapevine 1 (Steps 11, inset, and 12) for 4 reps, then step sideways with your right foot, cross back with your left, and sideways again with your right. Lift your left heel up as you snap the fingers of your right hand high up toward the ceiling. Repeat to the other side (shown here) for a total of 4 reps.

pressure on the ball of the foot

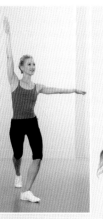

19 Step touch 2
Repeat Step touch 1 (Steps 13, inset, and 14) for 8 reps, then touch the toes of your right foot out to the right side, bring your right shoulder forward, and snap your fingers straight down toward the floor. Step your right foot back to center and square off your shoulders to prepare for the other side (shown here). Do 8 reps.

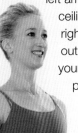

20 Ball change 3
Repeat Ball change 2 (Step 15, inset) for 4 reps, then cross your left foot back, reach your left arm up to the ceiling and your right arm straight out to the right. Lift your right foot and place it back on the floor. Bring your left foot back beneath you and your arms down by your sides, jumping in place before starting the other side. Do 4 reps.

accentuate the shoulders

legs together

point your toes

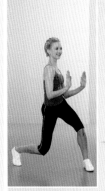

21 **Cross touch 3** Repeat Cross touch 2 (Step 16, inset) for 4 reps, then cross your left foot in front of your right. Bring your arms straight out at shoulder height as you step out on your right foot, then pick up and place down your left foot. Hop on that foot as you bend your right knee and touch it with your left hand. Cross your right foot in front of your left to repeat to the other side. Do a total of 4 reps.

strong arms

22 **Box step 3** Repeat Box step 2 (Step 17, inset) for 8 reps, then step forward on the right foot, bringing the left shoulder forward and flexing both hands. Then step the left foot forward, bring the right shoulder forward, and keep the hands flexed.

Quickly take two small jumps backward to your starting place while pushing away with both hands. Repeat 8 times.

point your toes

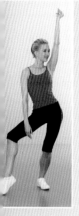

23 Grapevine 3 Repeat Grapevine 2 (Step 18, inset) for 4 reps. Then step sideways to the right, cross back to the left, and step sideways to the right again. Lift your heels up off the floor and reach both arms high to the ceiling. Stay on your toes as you bend your knees and drop your arms down toward the floor. Do 4 reps.

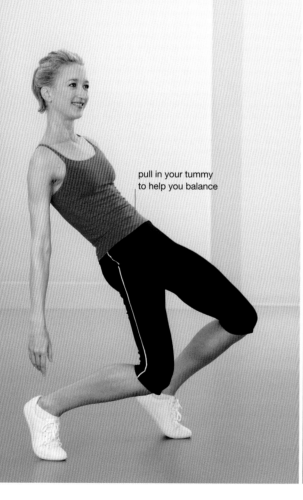

pull in your tummy to help you balance

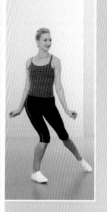

24 Step touch 3 Repeat Step touch 2 (Step 19, inset) for 8 reps. Then, starting with your feet together and your arms down by your sides, bend your right elbow as you jump. Now bring your right leg out to the side and place both heels down as you straighten your right arm and snap your fingers. Jump your feet back together and bring your arms down by your sides to repeat to the other side. Do a total of 8 reps.

Now repeat all the Level 3 steps, then repeat them again in reverse order. You have reached the height of your aerobic curve. To finish, repeat the entire sequence in reverse order, starting with Step 24, working back to Step 5, and cutting the number of reps in half to slowly bring your heart rate down.

>> **tone & stretch** abs/quads

25 **Abs** Lie on your back and lace your fingers behind your head with your knees bent and your feet hip-width apart. Inhale to prepare. As you exhale, lift your head off the floor using your abdominal muscles. Come up for 2 counts, and then relax for 2 counts. Repeat 4 times. Now repeat another 8 times, but this time quickly, using 1 count to come up and 1 count to go back down. Always lift your head off the mat using your abdominal muscles and your arms.

26 **Quads** Lie on your right side with your knees bent at a right angle in front of your body and your right arm out long. Relax your head on your outstretched right arm as you place your left hand on your left foot. Keeping your left leg parallel to the floor, gently pull your left foot behind you. Keep your back long as you stretch the front of your thigh.

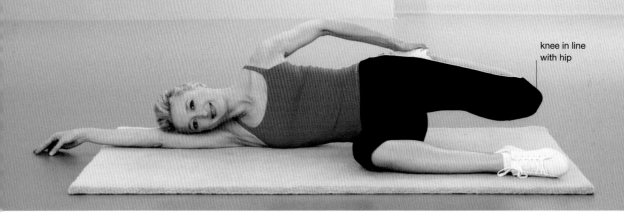

knee in line
with hip

27 **Spine** Place your left leg on top of your right and bring your arms straight out in front of your torso. Circle your left arm over your head, trying to keep your knees together and your hips square (inset). Then turn your head to follow your left hand and relax, stretching out both arms in opposite directions. Roll onto your left side and repeat Steps 26 and 27.

28 **Hamstrings** Lie on your back with your arms by your sides and your knees bent, feet flat on the floor and hip-width apart. Lengthen your right leg toward the ceiling and hold onto it comfortably with both hands. Breathing deeply, slowly bring your leg toward your chest, feeling a gentle stretch in the back of the extended leg. Repeat on the other side.

stretch the back of the thigh

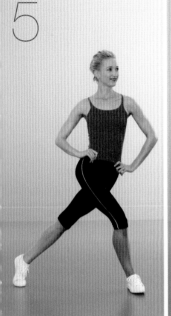

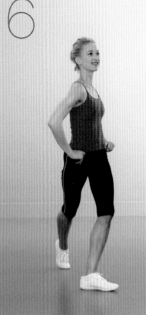

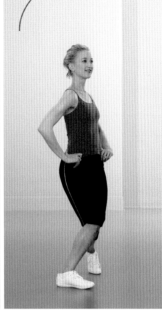

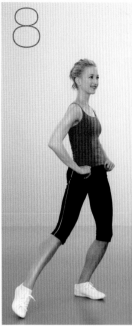

▲ **Aerobic** Ball change 1, page 70

▲ **Aerobic** Ball change 1, page 70

▲ **Aerobic** Cross touch 1, page 71

▲ **Aerobic** Cross touch 1, page 71

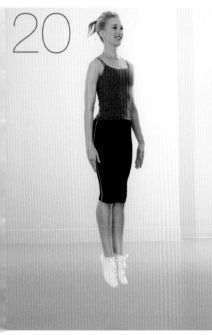

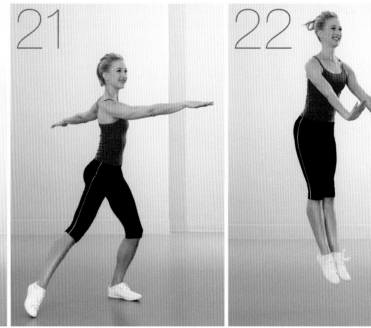

▲ **Aerobic** Ball change 3, page 77

▲ **Aerobic** Cross touch 3, page 78

▲ **Aerobic** Box step 3, page 78

jazz at a glance

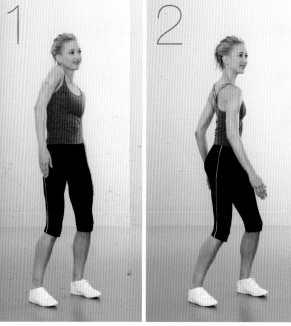

1
▲ **Warm-up** Plié shoulder circles, page 68

2
▲ **Warm-up** Torso twist, page 68

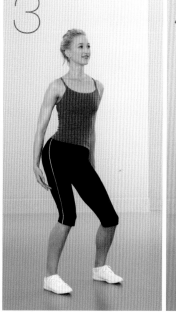

3
▲ **Warm-up** Hip side to side, page 69

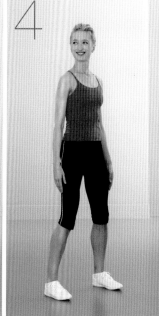

4
▲ **Warm-up** Head looks, page 69

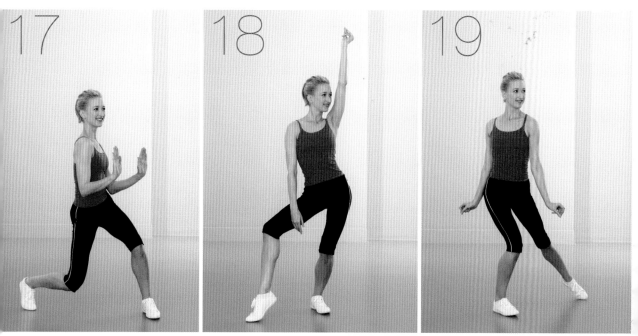

17
▲ **Aerobic** Box step 2, page 76

18
▲ **Aerobic** Grapevine 2, page 76

19
▲ **Aerobic** Step touch 2, page 77

jazz >>

>> **jazz** FAQs

The Jazz workout strengthens the heart and lungs while accentuating the hands, shoulders, and hips. Be sure to keep all of the accents and flair of the workout as the movements get more demanding. Imagine you are Liza Minnelli in *Cabaret*. If you're not feeling very "jazzy," here are a few pointers to get your fingers snapping!

What work does the Grapevine do?

It is a coordination exercise. Needing to move your feet, arms, and shoulders and do the snap all at the same time forces you to multitask, which is good exercise for your brain. These moves also add greater depth to the step. What is more, the Grapevine raises the heart rate and warms up the body. Be sure to travel side to side as much as possible while performing the movement. This will make your legs, heart, and lungs work harder.

I'm finding it difficult to stay in time with the music on Cross touch 1. Any tips?

Yes. Practice, practice, and practice! Start out practicing the movement slowly on its own. Then, try to pick up the pace a few times. When you're feeling ready, try the movements again, with the music. If you break down the step in this way, you will be dancing to the rhythm of the music in no time.

I find I am able to do the workout, but not all the jumps. Is this normal or should I be worried?

It's fine. Everyone starts out in different places. Some people have had dance experience, others might be runners with no dance training, while some might even be exercising for the first time. The important thing is not to judge yourself while you are learning something new. Always start with an open mind, a willingness to learn, and an eagerness to have fun.

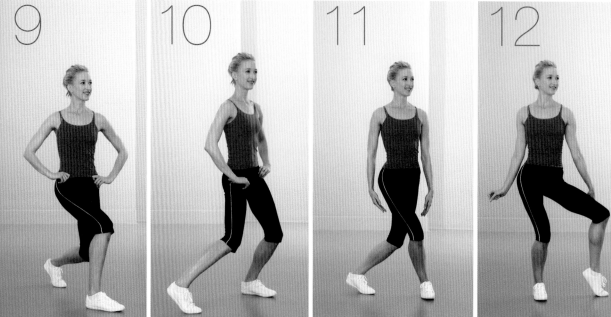

▲ **Aerobic** Box step 1, page 72

▲ **Aerobic** Box step 1, page 72

▲ **Aerobic** Grapevine 1, page 73

▲ **Aerobic** Grapevine 1, page 73

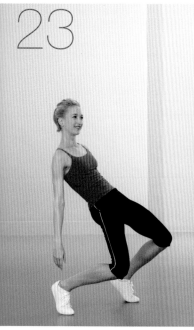

▲ **Aerobic** Grapevine 3, page 79

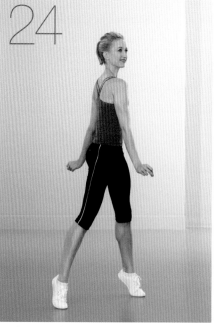

▲ **Aerobic** Step touch 3, page 79

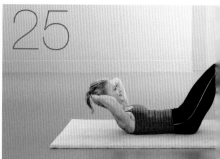

▲ **Tone & stretch**
Abs, page 80

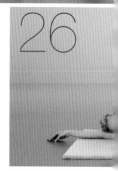

▲ **Tone & stretch**
Quads, page 80

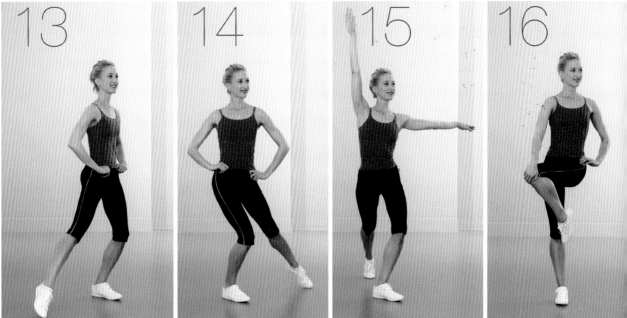

▲ **Aerobic** Step touch 1, page 74

▲ **Aerobic** Step touch 1, page 74

▲ **Aerobic** Ball change 2, page 75

▲ **Aerobic** Cross touch 2, page 75

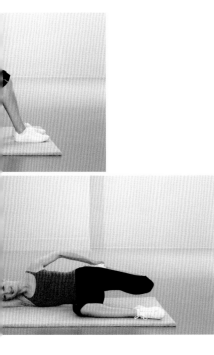

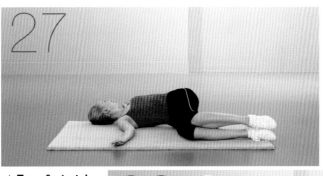

▲ **Tone & stretch** Spine, page 81

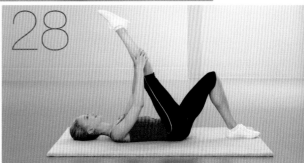

▲ **Tone & stretch** Hamstrings, page 81

15 minute **summary**

The arms on Ball change 2 and 3 are difficult. Can I just leave my hands on my hips?

Yes, but then your arms are missing a great opportunity to strengthen while lengthening. Keep trying the steps with the arms, making your arms sharp and long with the beat of the music. Focus on having fun rather than on how "perfect" the movement looks and, with practice, you will soon see an improvement in your coordination. And don't be afraid to go to the next level!

How do I control the drop on Grapevine 3?

First, think of all the movements in your body originating from your center—the abdominal muscles exert the control for all the outer movement. Pull your tummy muscles in as you lift up onto your toes with both arms reaching up to the ceiling. Then, as your arms fall toward the floor, your knees bend, and your heels come off the floor, pull your abdominal muscles in to control your balance. Try to do the drop with a small bend in the knees at first. As you gain confidence, you can bend your knees more.

The back of my legs are extremely tight. Is there any way to improve this?

Stretching on a regular basis will improve the tightness in the back of the thighs, or hamstrings. If you can, try to stretch your legs daily, even if just for a few minutes. Stretch slowly, allowing the muscles to relax into the stretch. If you spend a few minutes stretching every day, you will see results in no time.

I'm having trouble with the coordination of the hands and feet in Box step 2.

This step is intricate and fast, so break it down and do it slowly. First, try walking two steps forward and two steps backward, bringing the opposite hands forward and backward. Once you have mastered that movement, add in the arms. Next add a deep bend in the knees, as you are moving forward. Finally, when the movement feels more natural, try it in time with the music.

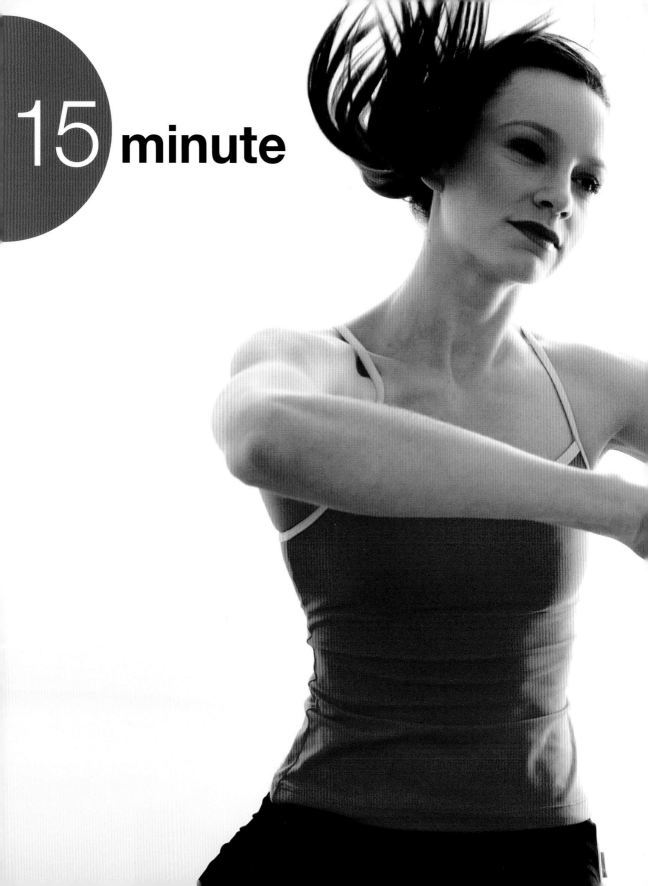

15 minute

Powerful. Grounded.
Precise. Funky. Learn
to dance with attitude.

street
workout >>

>> **warm-up** shoulder shrugs/shoulder circles

1 **Shoulder shrugs** With your feet hip-width apart and parallel, bend your knees over your toes. As you straighten your legs, point your right foot and tap the floor, lifting your shoulders toward your ears. Place your foot back and bend your knees to get ready for the other side (shown here). Repeat, alternating sides for 8 reps (1 rep = both sides).

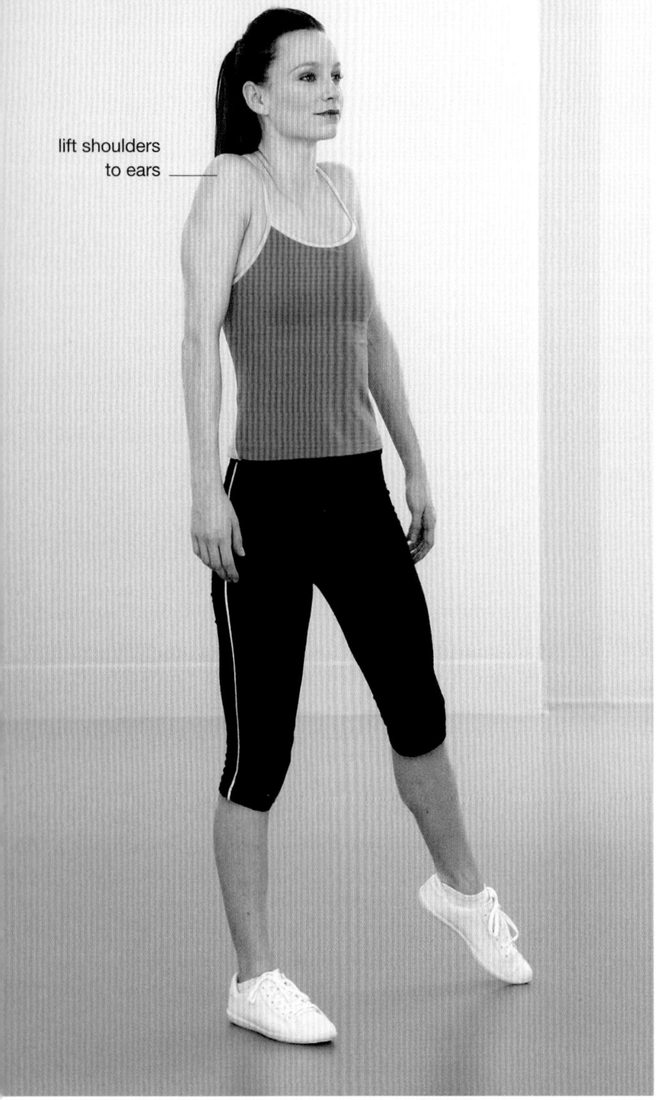

lift shoulders to ears

2 **Shoulder circles** Continue bending your knees and tapping your toes on the floor, but now add a shoulder circle forward to each tap. Repeat 8 times forward, then 8 times back.

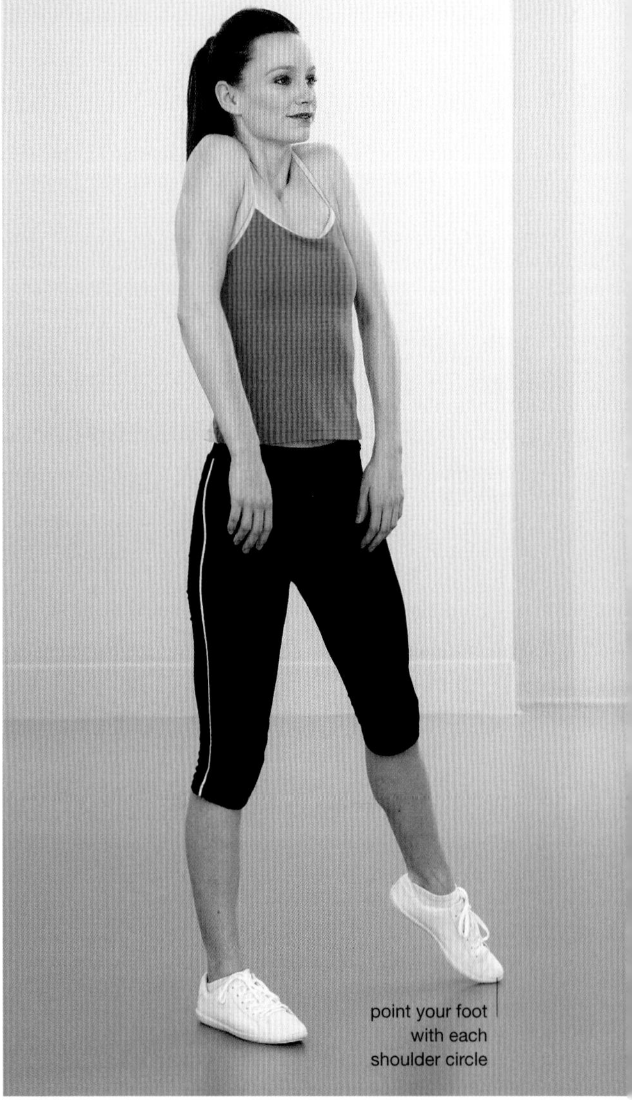

point your foot with each shoulder circle

3 **Side bends** Keep your feet on the floor, hip-width apart and parallel to each other. Starting from the top of your head, slowly bend directly sideways to your right. Let your left hand slide up to your ribs as your right hand slides down toward your knee. Come back to center and repeat to the other side. Do 2 reps.

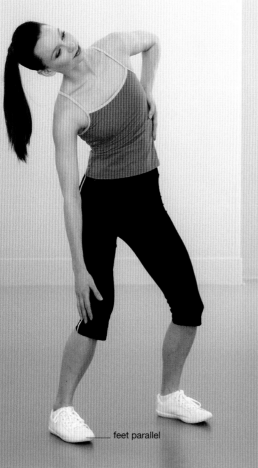

feet parallel

4 **Head looks** Straighten your knees and lengthen through the top of your head toward the ceiling. Look over your right shoulder. Bring your head back to center, then look over your left shoulder. Do 4 reps.

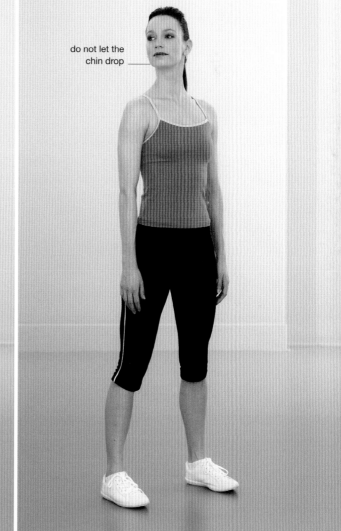

do not let the chin drop

>> **aerobic** box step 1

5 **Box step 1** Place your hands on your hips and bring your feet together. Then step forward and slightly out to the right side on your right foot.

6 Now step forward and slightly to your left side on your left foot. Then step back on your right foot, bringing it back to your starting position. Finish by bringing your left foot back to your right. Repeat Steps 5 and 6 for a total of 8 reps.

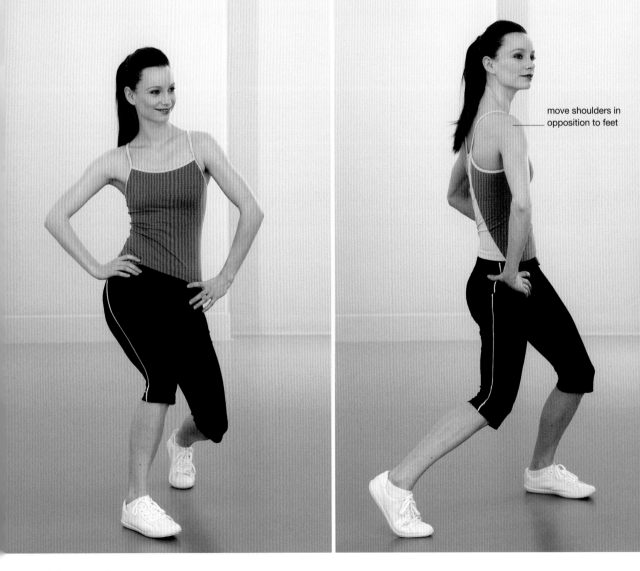

move shoulders in opposition to feet

7 **Hamstring curls 1** Place your hands on your hips as you step on your right foot. Bend your left knee slightly behind you, lengthening your left foot toward your bottom. Keep your navel pulled into your spine so that your back stays lengthened.

8 Place your left foot back onto the floor so that your feet are hip-width apart and your knees are soft. Repeat to the other side. Repeat Steps 7 and 8 for a total of 8 reps.

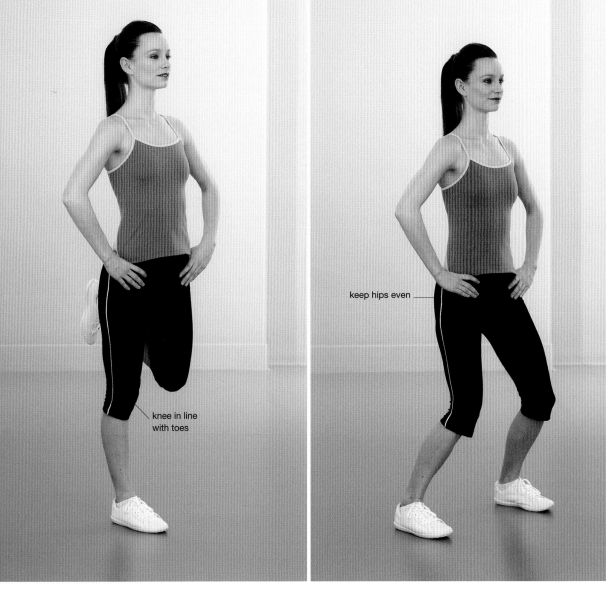

keep hips even

knee in line
with toes

>> **aerobic** grapevine 1

9 **Grapevine 1** Relax your arms by your sides with your hands near your hips. Take a small step to the side with your right foot.

10 Cross your left foot behind your right, lift your right, and take another small step to the right. Then lift your left foot and touch the toes of your left foot on the floor next to your right. Repeat to the left, starting with a step to the side with the left foot. Repeat Steps 9 and 10 for a total of 4 reps.

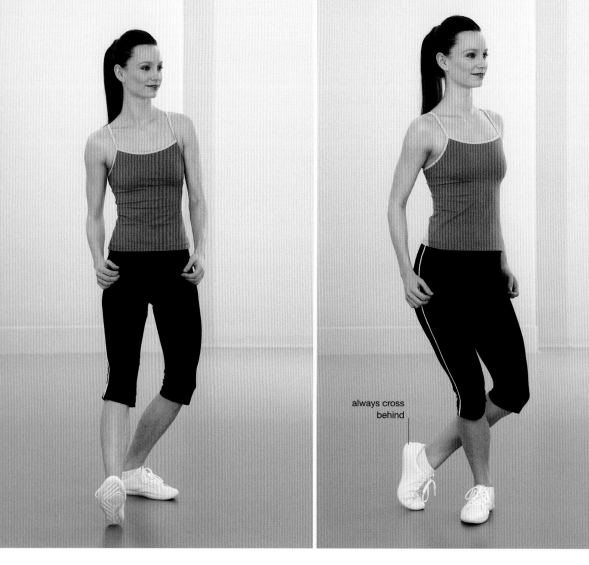

always cross behind

11 **Forward & back 1** Relax your arms down by your sides and walk forward, starting on your right foot. Walk three steps forward, and then bring your left foot to touch next to your right.

12 Then walk three steps backward and bring your right foot to touch next to your left. Keep your shoulders open and your head lengthening toward the ceiling. Repeat Steps 11 and 12 for a total of 4 reps.

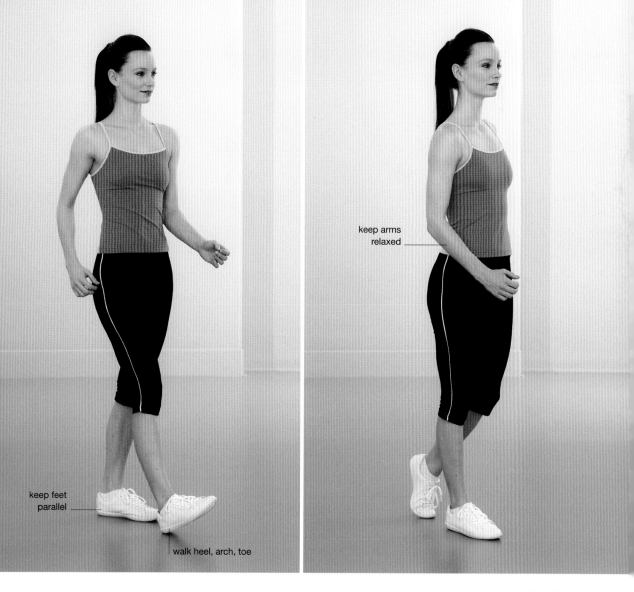

keep arms relaxed

keep feet parallel

walk heel, arch, toe

>> **aerobic** heel dig 1

13 **Heel dig 1** Take a tiny step beneath you with your right foot, then cross your left foot in front of your right, and "dig" the heel of your left foot on the floor.

14 Bring your left foot back onto the floor hip-width apart from your right foot, then repeat to the other side. Repeat Steps 13 and 14 for a total of 8 reps.

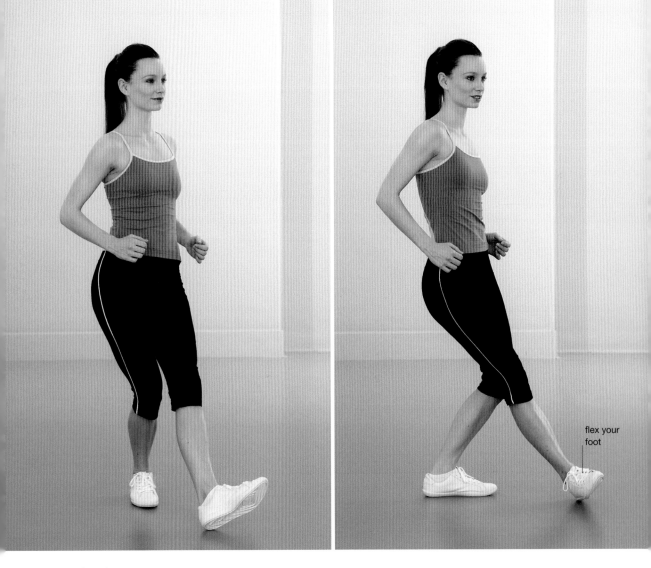

flex your foot

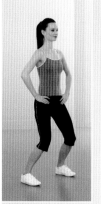

15 **Box step 2** Repeat Box step 1 (Steps 5, inset, and 6) for 8 reps. Step forward with your right foot, bringing your left shoulder and arm forward, then step forward and sideways with your left foot, bringing your right shoulder and arm forward (shown here). Now step back with your right foot, then with your left, alternating feet and shoulders. Do a total of 8 reps.

16 **Hamstring curls 2** Repeat Hamstring curls 1 (Steps 7 and 8, inset) for 8 reps, then step on your right foot and lift your left knee while raising your left elbow in front of you and your right elbow to the side. Repeat to the other side (shown here) for 8 reps.

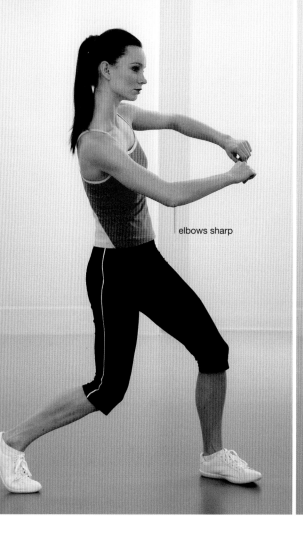

elbows sharp

keep hips level

arms form a box parallel to the ground

17 Grapevine 2
Repeat Grapevine 1 (Steps 9, inset, and 10) for 4 reps, then step sideways on your right foot, cross back with your left, and sideways again with your right. Now, instead of bringing in your left foot to touch, flex it and do a heel dig while lifting your shoulders and letting your hips swing forward. Repeat to the other side (shown here), then alternate sides for another 3 reps.

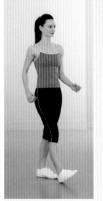

18 Forward & back 2
Repeat Forward & back 1 (Steps 11, inset, and 12) for 4 reps, then jog 3 steps forward and step together. Jog 3 steps back and step together. When jogging, roll through your feet and keep your knees soft. Repeat 3 more times.

roll through your foot ——————
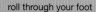

19 **Heel dig 2** Repeat Heel dig 1 (Steps 13, inset, and 14) for 8 reps, then relax your arms by your sides and step on your right foot. As you cross your left foot in front of your right for the dig, bend your elbows and raise your shoulders slightly up and back as you lift your hips forward. Relax your arms back by your sides as you place your left foot down to repeat to the other side (shown here). Alternate sides for a total of 8 reps.

strong arms

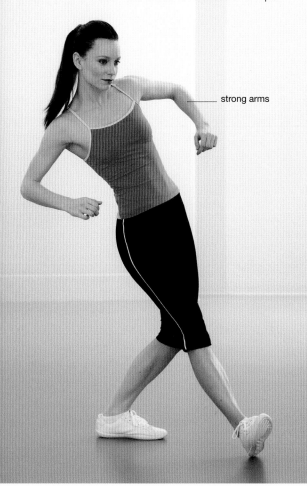

20 **Box step 3** Repeat Box step 2 (Step 15, inset) for 8 reps, then step forward on your right foot, bringing your left shoulder and arm forward. Then step forward on your left foot, with your right shoulder and arm coming forward. Finally, make 2 small jumps backward to your starting position. Repeat 8 times.

point your toes

>> **aerobic** hamstring curls 3/grapevine 3

21 Hamstring curls 3

Repeat Hamstring curls 2 (Step 16, inset) for 8 reps, then bend your left leg and jump softly onto your right as you swing your right elbow out to the side and bring your left elbow forward. Then jump off your right leg and place both feet back on the floor, hip-width apart, as your arms swing down to repeat on the other side. Do a total of 8 reps.

breathe fully and deeply

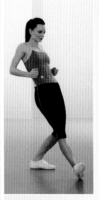

22 Grapevine 3

Repeat Grapevine 2 (Step 17, inset) for 4 reps, then, starting with your right foot, step sideways, crossing back with your left, and sideways again with your right. Now do a small hop and bring your left foot in to meet your right. Repeat, starting with your left foot, for a total of 4 reps.

accentuate the hop with the arms

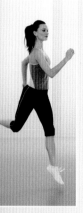

23 Forward & back 3

Repeat Forward & back 2 (Step 18, inset) for 4 reps, then jog forward, starting with your right foot, then left, right, and feet together. Now step sideways with your right foot, bringing your right elbow out to the side and your left elbow up in front. Step your feet together, then bring your left foot sideways, your right elbow in front, and your left elbow to the side (shown here). Jog back, starting on the right. Repeat one more time.

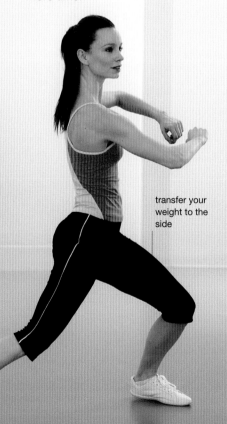

transfer your weight to the side

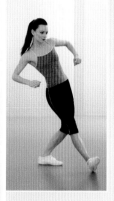

24 Heel dig 3

Repeat Heel dig 2 (Step 19, inset) for 8 reps, then lift your left knee. Bring both arms to the center of your body, then cross your left leg in front of your right and do a heel dig with your elbows out to the side. Bring your left knee back up and your arms back to center, then place your left foot down on the floor to repeat on the other side (shown here). Do a total of 4 reps.

Now repeat all the Level 3 steps, then repeat them again in reverse order.
You have reached the height of your aerobic curve. To finish, repeat the entire sequence in reverse order, starting with Step 24, working back to Step 5, and cutting the number of reps in half to bring your heart rate slowly back to rest.

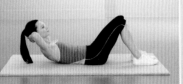

25 **Abs** Lie on your back and lace your fingers behind your head with your knees bent, feet flat on the floor and hip-width apart. Inhale to prepare. As you exhale, lift your head off the floor using your abdominal muscles (inset). Come up for 2 counts, then relax for 2 counts. Repeat 8 times, then lift your head center, stay high, and twist to the right. Come back to center and relax down. Repeat to the other side. Do 4 reps.

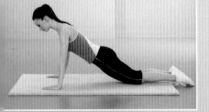

26 **Push-ups** Roll over onto your hands and knees. Place your hands beyond shoulder width and take your hips forward so that your shoulders, knees, and hips are all in one line (inset). Inhale as you bend your elbows straight out to the side; exhale as you straighten your arms. Repeat 8 times, always keeping your body in one straight line.

keep your back long

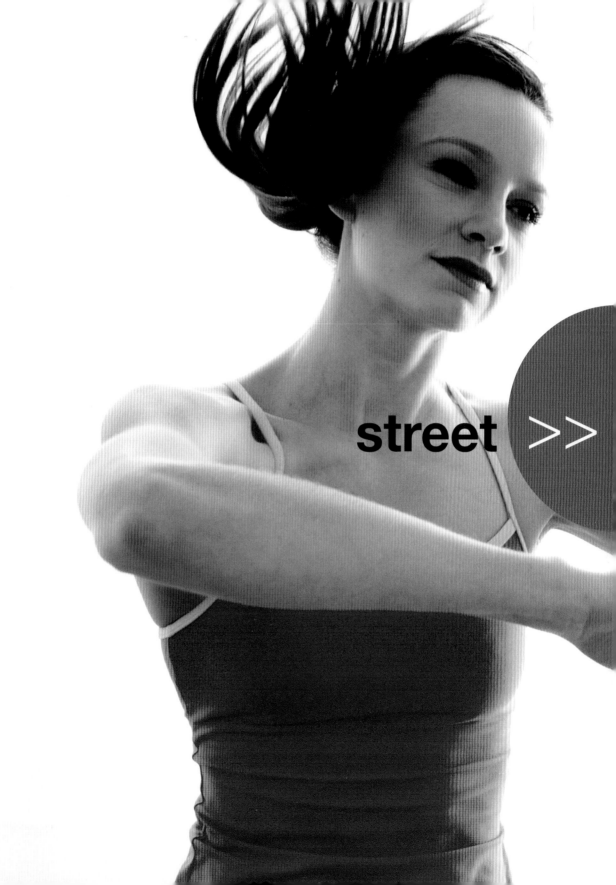

street >>

street at a glance

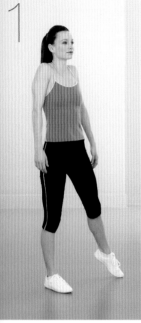

▲ **Warm-up** Shoulder shrugs, page 92

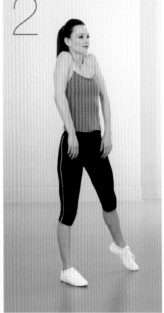

▲ **Warm-up** Shoulder circles, page 92

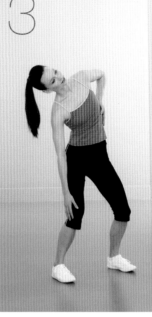

▲ **Warm-up** Side bends, page 93

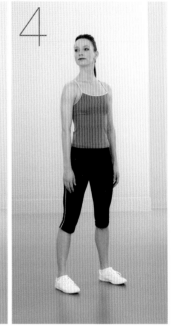

▲ **Warm-up** Head looks, page 93

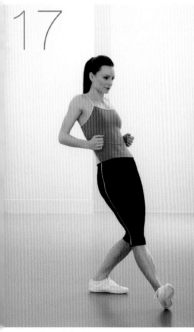

▲ **Aerobic** Grapevine 2, page 100

▲ **Aerobic** Forward & back 2, page 100

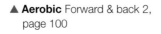

▲ **Aerobic** Heel dig 2, page 101

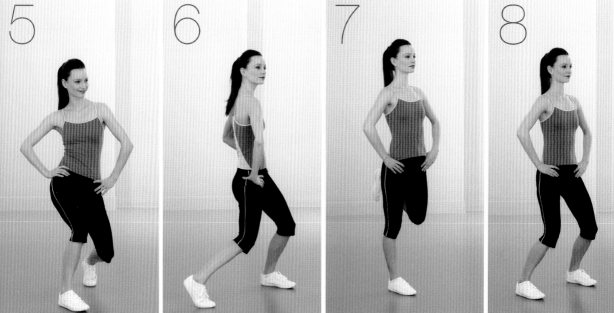

▲ **Aerobic** Box step 1, page 94

▲ **Aerobic** Box step 1, page 94

▲ **Aerobic** Hamstring curls 1, page 95

▲ **Aerobic** Hamstring curls 1, page 95

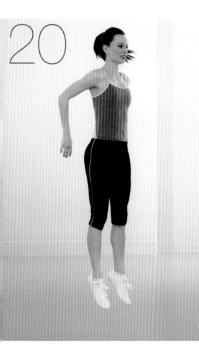

▲ **Aerobic** Box step 3, page 101

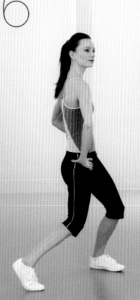

▲ **Aerobic** Hamstring curls 3, page 102

▲ **Aerobic** Grapevine 3, page 102

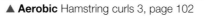
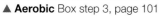

27 **Hips** Sit up with your legs straight out in front of you and together. Cross your left ankle above your right knee, then place your hands behind you and bend your right leg so your right foot is on the floor. Push your bottom forward and lift your chest so that you feel a stretch in your left hip. Relax and breathe.

28 **Thighs** Stretch both legs out, then bend your left leg, bringing the sole of your left foot to touch the right leg. Place both hands on your right leg and lengthen forward out of your back so that you feel a stretch in the back of your right leg. Relax and breathe, then repeat Steps 27 and 28 to the other side.

stretch the back of the thigh

>> **street** FAQs

The Street workout is sharp and funky. Bend your knees and isolate your hips, shoulders, head, and elbows. Play with each movement to make it your own—you might want to add one shoulder instead of two in places, or a flick of the hip where there isn't one. If you're not feeling very funky, here are some tips to help you get into the groove.

 ### I'm doing all the steps but I don't feel like I look very "street." Why is that?

Usually, when we move, we do so from the center of the body. Street dance has a very earthy feel, so think about having a lower center of gravity when performing this workout. To do this, imagine your weight being lower in the body and move more from your hips and legs.

>> What exactly should my shoulders and hips be doing in Grapevine 2?

At the end of the movement, as you flex your foot and do a heel dig, you want to let your shoulders swing back and up as if you were shrugging. As you do this, let your hips swing forward as though you are tucking your pelvis slightly underneath yourself.

 ### I feel so uncoordinated in Heel digs 3. Any tips?

Again, practice, practice, and more practice. Heel digs 3 should be a great, fun move. Read the explanatory text on p103 and go through the move carefully. Practice the coordination on both sides. Then, slowly build up so you move faster and faster. Part of the fun in learning something new is the accomplishment of your goals.

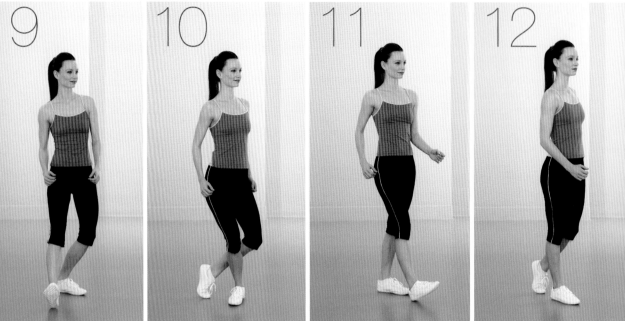

▲ **Aerobic** Grapevine 1,
page 96

▲ **Aerobic** Grapevine 1,
page 96

▲ **Aerobic** Forward & back 1,
page 97

▲ **Aerobic** Forward & back 1,
page 97

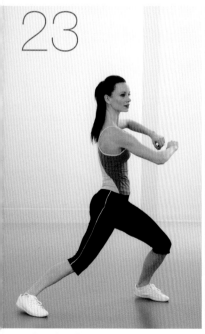

▲ **Aerobic** Forward & back 3,
page 103

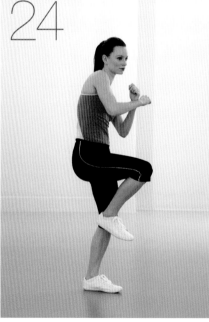

▲ **Aerobic** Heel dig 3, page 103

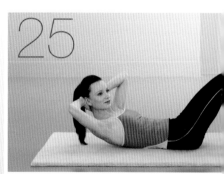

▲ **Tone & stretch**
Abs, page 104

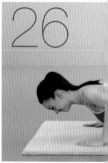

▲ **Tone & stretch** P

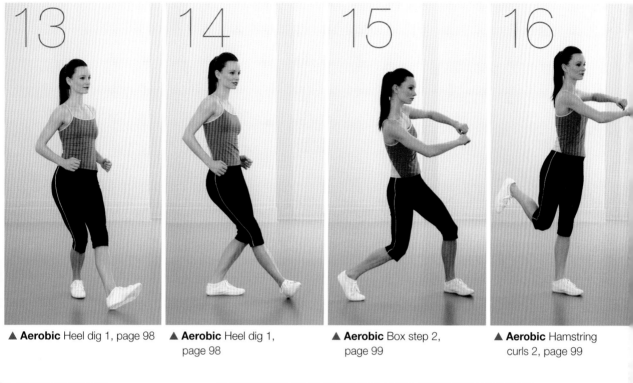

▲ **Aerobic** Heel dig 1, page 98

▲ **Aerobic** Heel dig 1, page 98

▲ **Aerobic** Box step 2, page 99

▲ **Aerobic** Hamstring curls 2, page 99

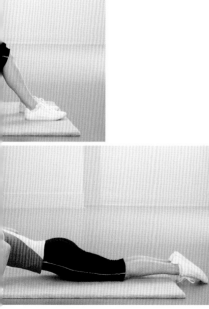

sh-ups, page 104

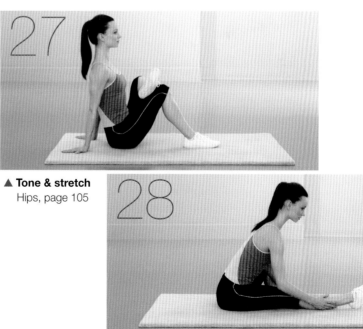

▲ **Tone & stretch** Hips, page 105

▲ **Tone & stretch** Thighs, page 105

15 minute **summary**

>> **I don't understand the opposition of the shoulders and feet in Box step 1, 2, and 3. Any suggestions?**

First, analyze how you walk normally. Do you notice how your shoulders move in slight opposition to the foot you are stepping on? The Box step is nothing more than an overexaggeration of this normal phenomenon.

>> **Is it OK if I stick to the second variation of each movement and never do the third?**

Yes, but only if you are working at your maximum level of fitness. It is your workout, and you know your body and your level of fitness best. But if you are doing the second variation and know that you can do the third, then you should definitely push for the third.

>> **I find it extremely difficult to keep my back straight in Push-ups. Is there a modification I can do?**

You should always make sure your back is flat in this exercise. If you can't achieve this, stay on your hands and knees with the hips back, and simply aim your nose just beyond your hands. When your muscles get stronger, try the variation (inset, Step 26, p104), using just a very small range of motion. Then, when you are ready, do the full exercise (Step 26, p104).

>> **What are my arms supposed to be doing in Hamstring curls 2 and 3?**

Think of your elbows as accenting the beat of the music. Make soft fists with your hands and a strong box shape with your arms. Lean into the movement as your knee bends behind you.

15 minute

dance
roundup >>

Tying it all together: Some dance terms and styles, and tips for when you are ready to progress and find a class.

>> **glossary** of dance terms

As you perform the dance workouts in this fitness program, you will come across some dance terms that may not be familiar to you. These pages are designed to help you understand them better. Always start with your feet together and parallel, unless stated otherwise.

Attitude Start with your feet hip-width apart and your knees soft. Take your right knee to hip height, making sure the knee is at a right angle. Place the right foot down and repeat on the left side.

Ball change Cross your right foot behind your left, lift the left foot briefly, and take your right shoulder slightly forward. Bring the right foot back, then repeat on the other side, taking the left shoulder forward when the left foot is behind.

The photographs below and opposite illustrate some basic ballet terms, as used in the Ballet workout.

Box step Take a big step forward with your right foot, then step sideways with your left. Step back with your right foot, then bring your left foot back.

Cross forward Cross your right foot in front of your left and step on it. Bring your right foot back to its starting position and repeat on the other side.

Cross touch Cross your right foot in front of your left and step on it, then bring your left foot to the side, touching your toes to the floor. Now cross your left foot in front of your right to repeat on the other side. This step is repeated moving both forward and backward.

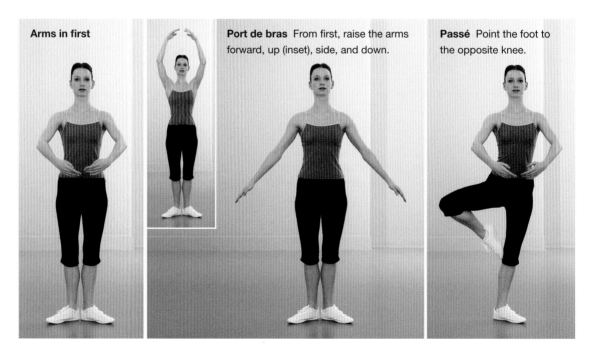

Arms in first

Port de bras From first, raise the arms forward, up (inset), side, and down.

Passé Point the foot to the opposite knee.

Double side step Step your right foot sideways, then bring your left foot to meet your right. Repeat to the right again, then repeat the whole sequence to the left. Let the hips rise and fall.

Grapevine Step to the side with your right foot, then cross your left foot behind your right, and step on it. Step sideways again with your right foot, this time bringing your left foot to meet the right. Repeat on the other side.

Hamstring curls Start with your feet hip-width apart and your knees soft. Bend your right knee, taking your right foot toward your buttocks. Then place your right foot down, and bend your left knee, taking your left foot toward your buttocks.

Mambo Cross the right foot in front of the left, rock onto your toes, lift the left foot, and place it back. Bring your right foot diagonally back to the right, rock onto your toes, and again lift the left foot and place it back. Repeat crossing the right foot in front of the left, the rock and the lift of the left foot, then take three small steps, starting with the right. Repeat on the other side, starting with your left foot.

Prances Start with heels together, toes slightly apart. Come onto your toes with straight legs. As you slowly lower the left foot back to the ground, bend your right knee so that you are still on the ball of your right foot. Then, come back up onto your toes and change sides by slowly lowering the right foot back to the ground and bending your left knee.

Salsa Start with your hands on your hips. Take a small step forward with the right foot, letting the right hip swing sideways. Then bring the right foot center and repeat, taking a small step forward with the left foot and letting the left hip swing. Bring the left foot center, then step back on the right foot, and center. Then back with the left foot, and center.

Step touch Touch the toes of the right foot out to the side, then bring the foot back to center. Repeat on the other side. As you step one foot out, swing the same shoulder forward and the opposite shoulder back.

Side lunge Take your right foot sideways, and bring your right shoulder forward as you rock onto your right toes, lifting your left foot briefly. Bring your right foot back to center. Repeat on the other side.

Toe taps Start with the feet in Second position (see below), then softly bend the knees, transfer your weight to the left foot, straighten the right leg, and tap the toes of the right foot on the floor. Bend both knees again and repeat on the other side.

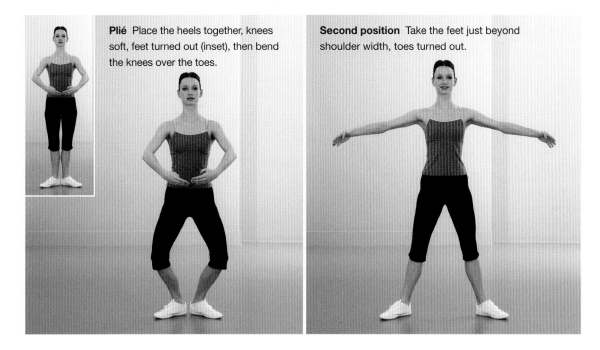

Plié Place the heels together, knees soft, feet turned out (inset), then bend the knees over the toes.

Second position Take the feet just beyond shoulder width, toes turned out.

>> **dance** styles

This *15-minute Dance Workout* program gives you the chance to experience four different dance styles. Each has its own flavor and technique, and each offers something slightly different in terms of musicality and how you move the parts of your body.

Salsa has a sensuous feel, with its gentle rolling of the hips and wrists. Ballet lengthens and elongates the muscles while teaching poise and grace. Jazz dance is strong, with fast and sharp footwork and arms. Street dance, with its musical score accenting the down beat, helps to ground us.

Naturally, you will feel more comfortable with some forms of dance than with others, but it is extremely important to practice all of them. Being open to trying new things keeps you young, healthy, free-spirited, and spontaneous. It also helps you to rediscover the child in you. So turn up the music and have some fun!

Salsa

Salsa is an exhilarating and vibrant way to stay in shape. It is also great for boosting your confidence, both on and off the dance floor. The foot patterns are simple to learn, and adding on the "salsa elements"—the movements of the hips, wrists, and shoulders—is sexy and fun. Rolling the wrists and placing the hands near the body can be sensuous and alluring. The hips should be relaxed and should swing gracefully with the movement of the feet. The subtle movements you make with your shoulders highlight the feel and rhythm of the music.

This enjoyable, flirtatious dance style traces its origins and influences back through many Latin and Afro-Caribbean cultures. Salsa originally started in Cuba, where there was a blending of different ethnic populations with immigrants from Europe and Africa. Spanish troubadours, Africans with their

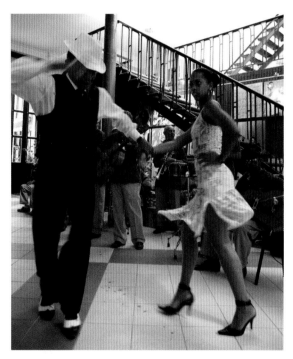

Salsa dancers in a café in Havana. Salsa is often performed in local venues such as cafés, clubs, restaurants, and halls.

drumbeats, and the native Cubans all created the music we know today as salsa. While Cuba is considered the birthplace of salsa, the name itself was actually invented much later in the 1970s—in New York City. Puerto Ricans and African-Americans have also had a major influence on salsa. The foundation of salsa is a rhythmic pattern called the clave. The most common clave is the son clave, which is characterized by three notes in the first bar and two in the second.

In my Salsa workout, I include several steps from dance styles with similar Latin-American origins to salsa. The steps for salsa and mambo, for example, are six steps over an eight-count phrase (see p17). This sounds more difficult than it is, but the trick is to first follow the steps made by the feet. Once you are comfortable with the movements of the feet, let the hips swing with the rhythm and the shoulders move quietly on top. Then add the arms and let the rhythm take over!

Ballet

The graceful movements of ballet have appealed to audiences and dancers alike for centuries. For the dancer, ballet technique gives poise, grace, elegance, and beauty. It also instills proper alignment, which carries over into excellent posture in everyday life. How you carry yourself is at the heart of ballet. While training, you are constantly lifting up out of your center. With every movement, you are thinking of lengthening your head to the ceiling while extending away through your heels. It is impossible to stand beautifully in ballet and then slouch through the rest of your day. Ballet lifts you up and invigorates your body as well as your soul.

Classical ballet was first performed in the royal courts of Renaissance Italy. The elaborate spectacles held there included dancing, music, and poetry. Originally, the dances were very simple in both plot and movement. Soon, the popularity of these spectacles caught on in France, where the dancing style became more intricate. Now the dancers would form lines and patterns that could best be seen by audiences from above.

At first, men performed all the roles, wearing masks and wigs while portraying females. By the

Tamara Rojo as Juliet and Carlos Acosta as Romeo. Notice the length and energy through the dancers' legs and feet, coupled with their soft, graceful arms.

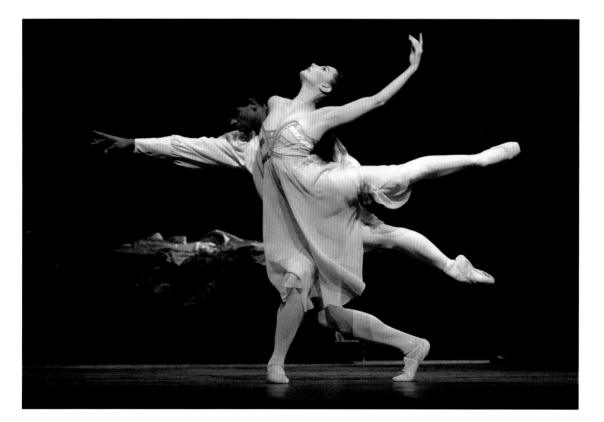

eighteenth century, women were dancing, too, and wearing large hoop skirts. Later, the skirts were shortened so the audience could appreciate the impressive footwork.

By the end of the eighteenth century, the ballet had spread to Vienna, where dancers and directors began exploring the use of dramatic themes and appropriate accompanying gestures. As the art form grew in popularity, there were further developments. For example, in 1796, the choreographer Charles Didelot, who worked in England and Russia, was the first person to attach invisible wires to the dancers to make them appear to fly. Dancing on the toes made its appearance soon after, but dancers would only dance on their toes for a few seconds.

The romantic ballet began in the 1830s with the ballet *La Sylphide*, which tells a story of supernatural and doomed love. The most famous ballets of the romantic repertoire were created during the rest of the nineteenth century.

Since the twentieth century, the breadth and scope of ballet has continued to increase, and ballet can now be found all over the world. There are also many dance forms that have developed from ballet, including modern dance—sometimes referred to as contemporary dance—jazz, and tap.

Jazz dance

This is a lively and playful dance form, with "sharp" shoulders and finger snaps. It brings to mind cigar bars, saxophones, late nights, and girls dressed in high heels and glamorous clothes. The history and style of jazz dance is completely intertwined with the music, so it is virtually impossible to describe one without the other.

Jazz dance emerged after World War I, although the music originated earlier, at the end of the nineteenth century in the US in New Orleans, St. Louis, and Memphis. The music flourished in the 1920s and brought with it a blossoming of cabarets and night clubs. It was then that the term "flapper" was coined. This referred to a new generation of women who had their hair cut in a bob, sported short skirts, listened to jazz and

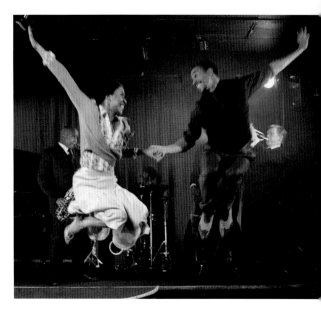

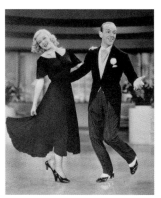

Jazz dance covers a wide spectrum of choreography, ranging from lyrical to sharp dance movements.

Ginger Rogers and Fred Astaire helped to bring jazz and musical theater into mainstream culture.

ragtime, and shunned social convention whenever possible. Flappers loved to dance the foxtrot, the shimmy, and the ever-famous Charleston.

Jazz music is a multicultural mix whose diverse origins include African, Spanish, French, English, German, and Italian. It is characterized by its syncopation, where the stress is on the weak beats in the musical phrase instead of on the strong beats. Another characteristic is its swing—a strong rhythm section played by the drums and double bass.

This new-fangled syncopation and swing were the ultimate rejection of the previous generation's light, romantic music. Until that point, musical phrasing had followed a set structure of beats and phrases, with the accent on the first and the third beat of a musical phrase. The obvious way to counter this was to stress the weaker beats—the second and the fourth.

Jazz dance, together with social convention, has changed enormously since the 1920s and the days of the flappers. During his 76 years in show business, renowned dancer, choreographer, and actor Fred Astaire made his own unique contribution to jazz by adding elements of ballet and ballroom dancing. Bob Fosse, the outstanding choreographer and musical theater director, and roughly contemporary with Fred Astaire, added a highly stylized sensuality and drama to theatrical jazz dance. Even today, jazz dance continues to change and grow as new choreographers emerge.

Street dance

This is a broad term used to describe modern dance characterized by funky beats, an earthy sound, and a loose form. It embraces a wide variety of dance styles including hip-hop, funk, house, and even break dancing. The routines performed in pop music videos are often a form of street dance. Personal style and improvisation are at its heart. Street dance can be performed anywhere, but is usually seen in clubs, at house parties, and in school yards. Informal groups gather and participants take turns improvising. Spontaneity, originality, and versatility are key. Informal competitions, called "battles," find individuals or groups dancing against each other in turns. The onlookers decide the winner.

Improvisation takes many forms. Dancers can move on the beat of the music, or on the off-beat. They can accent different aspects of the music by isolating and moving different body parts. They can keep the rhythm of the music with the feet, with the hips, or even just with one shoulder. The fun of street dance is its versatility. Anything goes! The important thing is to have fun and enjoy the beat.

Many grassroot dance companies such as the one below specialize in bringing popular dance culture into classical dance venues.

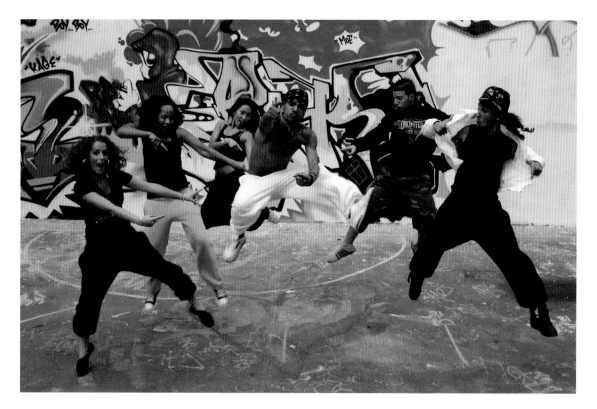

>> **finding** a class and teacher

Now that you have enjoyed a taste of the benefits of dance in your own home, chances are that you have become hooked enough to want to develop your newfound skills further. A dance class is a great way to learn more, improve your fitness levels, and have some fun.

It is important to find a class and instructor that are right for you. The best way is by recommendation from a friend or colleague. You can also try your local gym or, if they don't run dance classes, your library or town hall can provide you with a list of places that do. Watch out, too, for the many community outreach programs that exist to promote exercise. And, of course, the Internet is also an excellent way to find classes in your area.

Checking what is offered

When choosing where to go for your class, it is worth making a list of points that are important to you. Depending on your priorities, such a list might look like the one shown here (see right).

Once you have found a class, you need to see if the instructor is right for you. Check also that he or she is certified to teach the class. There are a wide variety of dance instructors with an enormous range of certifications, so take your time finding one. Don't be too shy to inquire about the training course the instructor has attended. Ideally, he or she will have taken a lengthy course (be wary of the instructor trained in one weekend) with both written and practical exams. Written tests are fine for assessing a person's knowledge, but practical exams should ensure that your teacher can communicate that knowledge in a clear, well-organized manner.

It is also important that, as well as your instructor being highly qualified, you feel a good rapport with him or her. If you do, you are more likely to attend classes regularly.

>> **points to look for** in a class

- **qualified, friendly** teacher?
- **classes that suit** your level of fitness?
- **convenient class times** that fit in with your daily activities?
- **price that** suits your pocket?
- **convenient location** and parking facilities?
- **comfortable,** clean surroundings?
- **clean** floor mats?
- **good changing facilities,** showers, and secure lockers?
- **towel rental** possible?
- **drinking water** freely available?
- **somewhere to** have a snack?
- **child care** if you need it?

And finally, notice if you like the atmosphere and feel positive about the class. Does the teacher make you feel welcome? Do you get enough individual attention? You may need to try several different classes until you find the one that works best for you. You should be looking for a class that makes your dance exercise fun and energizing.

Make sure you find a teacher who gives you individualized feedback in a friendly, positive atmosphere.

123

useful resources

Dance and fitness are ever-growing areas and, hopefully, you will now be inspired to explore them further. However, it is always best to do a little research before venturing off on new endeavors. Here are a few resources to help you get started when you feel ready to take things further, try something new, or get into a class.

dance resources

Dance Net Fitness
www.dancenetfitness.com
Find a dance studio near you.

Dance Sport UK
www.dancesport.uk.com/
studios_world/index.htm
List of dance studios worldwide.

Fitness USA
www.fitnessusa.com
Offers dance aerobics classes at neighborhood fitness centers throughout Michigan, Indiana, and California.

National Dance Week
www.nationaldanceweek.org
The Coalition for National Dance Week was formed in 1981 to bring greater recognition to dance as an art form across the United States.

Voice of Dance
www.voiceofdance.org
Offers a local class finder and global dance directory.

general fitness resources

About Aerobics
www.aboutaerobics.com
Website offering fitness advice, articles, and exercise tips.

Aerobic and Fitness Association of America (AFAA)
15250 Ventura Blvd., Suite 200
Sherman Oaks, CA 91403
www.afaa.com
Tel:1-877-YOUR-BODY
The world's largest fitness and TeleFitness® educator. Since 1983, AFAA has issued over 250,000 certifications to fitness professionals from more than 73 countries around the world.

American Council of Exercise (ACE)
4851 Paramount Drive
San Diego, CA 92123
www.acefitness.org
Tel: 1-888-825-3636
ACE is a nonprofit organization committed to enriching quality of life through safe and effective physical activity. ACE protects all segments of society against ineffective fitness products, programs, and trends through its ongoing public education, outreach and research. ACE further protects the public by setting certification and continuing education standards for fitness professionals.

American College of Sports Medicine (ACSM)
401 West Michigan Street
Indianapolis, IN 46202-3233
www.acsm.org
Tel: (317) 637-9200
ACSM promotes and integrates scientific research, education, and practical applications of sports medicine and exercise science to maintain and enhance physical performance, fitness, health, and quality of life.

IDEA Health & Fitness Association
10455 Pacific Center Court
San Diego, CA 92121-4339
Tel: (800) 999-4332, ext. 7
www.ideafit.com
An association of health and fitness professionals.

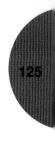

International Fitness Professional Association (IFPA)

14509 University Point Place
Tampa, FL 33613
Tel: (813) 979-1925
www.ifpa-fitness.com
Offers over 60 certifications and over 100 continuing education courses for Fitness, Health, Nutrition, Sports Conditioning, and Medical Professionals.

National Exercise Training Association (NETA)

5955 Golden Valley Rd, Suite 240
Minneapolis, MN 55422
Tel: 800-AEROBIC
www.netafit.org
NETA has certified over 120,000 fitness professionals and is recognized as a leader in the fitness industry. Its Certifications are recognized at over 18,000 fitness facilities across the US.

The American Physical Therapy Association

www.APTA.org
The mission of the American Physical Therapy Association (APTA), the principal membership organization representing and promoting the profession of physical therapy, is to further the profession's role in the prevention, diagnosis, and treatment of movement dysfunctions and the enhancement of the physical health and functional abilities of members of the public.

apparel

Adidas

610 Broadway,
New York, NY 10012
Phone: 212-5290081
www.adidas.com

Danskin®

530 Seventh Ave
New York, NY 10018
Tel: 1-800-288-6749
www.danskin.com

Lululemon

Union Square
327 Grant Avenue
San Francisco, CA 94108
Tel: (415) 402-0914
www.lululemon.com
Well-designed, comfortable clothes to work out and run around in, with stores in Canada, the US, Australia, and Japan

Nike (World Headquarters)

One Bowerman Drive
Beaverton, OR 97005
Tel: 1-503-671-6453
www.nike.com

Masai Barefoot Technology (MBT)

Masai USA Corp
515 North River Street, Unit D
Hailey, ID 83333
www.swissmasaius.com
Unique shoes to improve posture.

Foot Locker Inc. Headquarters

112 West 34th Street
New York, NY 10120
Tel: (212) 720-3700
www.footlocker.com

Reebok

Reebok International
1895 JW Foster Blvd.
Canton, MA 02021
Phone: 781-401-5000

other books by Caron Bosler

Healthy Inspiration: Yoga and Pilates –Total Body Workout
(D & S Books, 2006)
By combining Pilates exercises and Yoga asanas, it is easy to get a great workout.

Healthy Inspiration: Absolute Pilates
(D & S Books, 2005)
This book combines the original exercises of Joseph Pilates with the innovations of pioneer Alan Herdman, the first person to bring Pilates to the UK in 1971.

Healthy Inspiration: Massage
(D & S Books, 2005)
This book teaches basic massage techniques with step-by-step photographs so anyone can massage like a professional.

index

acknowledgments

Author's acknowledgments

I would sincerely like to thank some of the many people who have made this book possible. First, Alycea Ungaro for putting my name forward to do it, and second, my fabulous boyfriend and manager, Sven Lorenz, for pushing me when I hesitated; Jenny Latham for taking that crucial leap of faith in me, and for her wonderful support and encouragement throughout; Hilary Mandleberg for her fabulous eye, editorial expertise, and kindness; Anne Fisher for her positive approach to impossible situations, as well as for her beautiful layouts; Ruth Jenkinson, for her amazing photographs; Vic Barnes, for spectacular makeup and hair; everyone at Chrome Productions for their magical editing abilities and musical scores; all of my wonderful clients for their endless support, love, and advice in both work and play; and the beautiful dancer, Harriet Latham, who put endless hours, dedication, and Sundays into making this book possible.

Publisher's acknowledgments

Dorling Kindersley would like to thank photographer Ruth Jenkinson and her assistants Ann Burke and Nathan Jenkinson; sweatyBetty for the loan of some of the exercise clothing; Viv Riley at Touch Studios; the model Harriet Latham; and Victoria Barnes for the hair and makeup.

Picture credits

The publisher would like to thank the following for their kind permission to reproduce their photographs: Bettman/Corbis, p120 (bottom); Digital Vision/Alamy, p118 and p120 (top); Julia Grossi/zefa/Corbis, p121; Robbie Jack/Corbis, p119.

All other images © Dorling Kindersley
For further information, see www.dkimages.com

about Caron Bosler

Caron Bosler holds a Masters in Dance from Laban Contemporary Dance Centre, London, and was also on Merit Scholarship with The Merce Cunningham Dance Company. She has been certified by The Pilates Studio, NYC, and by Alan Herdman, London, is a registered member of the Pilates Foundation and of The Pilates Method Alliance, and is also certified in aerobics. As a dancer, Caron has performed with international choreographer Stephan Koplowitz, both in the US and, as part of Dance Umbrella, in England. She has also performed in "The English Ballet" in Casablanca, Morocco. In addition, Caron has choreographed throughout her dance career.

Her work includes "Gripping from the Inside" (1996), "Between Sound and Body" (1998), and "Un árbol que crece torcido nunca se endereza" (2001). She gives private lessons in aerobics and Pilates and, for her own enjoyment, attends dance classes at Pineapple Dance Studios and at Dance Works in London. Among Caron's other books are: *Healthy Inspiration: Absolute Pilates* and *Healthy Inspiration: Yoga and Pilates–Total Body Workout*.

Caron can be contacted via her website at www.caronboslerpilates.com or email caronbosler@pilatesinternational.com